MW01383384

**Practicing Psychology
in Primary Care**

About the Author

H. Russell Searight is Associate Professor of Psychology at Lake Superior State University in Sault Sainte Marie, Michigan. For 18 years, he was Director of Behavioral Science at the Forest Park Hospital Family Medicine Residency and on the faculty of Saint Louis University School of Medicine. He has published three previous books and over 140 articles and book chapters.

Practicing Psychology in Primary Care

H. Russell Searight

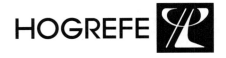

Library of Congress Cataloging in Publication

is available via the Library of Congress Marc Database under the
LC Control Number 2009938536

Library and Archives Canada Cataloguing in Publication

Searight, H. Russell
    Practicing psychology in primary care / H. Russell Searight.

Includes bibliographical references.
ISBN 978-0-88937-362-4

    1. Clinical psychology–Practice. 2. Psychology–Practice.
3. Primary health care. I. Title.

RC467.95.S42 2009   362.2   C2009-906175-9

PUBLISHING OFFICES
USA: Hogrefe Publishing, 875 Massachusetts Avenue, 7th Floor, Cambridge, MA 02139
            Phone (866) 823-4726, Fax (617) 354-6875; E-mail customerservice@hogrefe-publishing.com
EUROPE: Hogrefe Publishing, Rohnsweg 25, 37085 Göttingen, Germany
            Phone +49 551 49609-0, Fax +49 551 49609-88, E-mail publishing@hogrefe.com

SALES & DISTRIBUTION
USA: Hogrefe Publishing, Customer Services Department, 30 Amberwood Parkway,
            Ashland, OH 44805
            Phone (800) 228-3749, Fax (419) 281-6883, E-mail customerservice@hogrefe.com
EUROPE: Hogrefe Publishing, Rohnsweg 25, 37085 Göttingen, Germany
            Phone +49 551 49609-0, Fax +49 551 49609-88, E-mail publishing@hogrefe.com

OTHER OFFICES
CANADA: Hogrefe Publishing, 660 Eglinton Ave. East, Suite 119-514, Toronto, Ontario M4G 2K2
SWITZERLAND: Hogrefe Publishing, Länggass-Strasse 76, CH-3000 Bern 9

Hogrefe Publishing
Incorporated and registered in the Commonwealth of Massachusetts, USA, and in Göttingen, Lower Saxony,
Germany

Printed and bound in the USA
ISBN 978-0-88937-362-4

Table of Contents

Chapter 1

Introduction to Primary Care Psychology

A Day in the Life of a Primary Care Psychologist

6:30 a.m.

You are riding your exercise bicycle at home when your cell phone rings. The hospital unit clerk from Six North, a general medical floor, is on the phone indicating that a Dr. Johnson has requested that you see a patient in the hospital this morning. The patient, Ms. St. Laurent, is a 75-year-old White female who was admitted after falling at home. It was later determined that she had fractured her hip. Surgery is scheduled for this afternoon. However, late yesterday, she became increasingly confused and her thoughts disorganized. Given the planned surgery, nursing staff and the surgeon were concerned about whether or not she could give meaningful informed consent to the procedure. During the course of the night, she became increasingly agitated and described visual hallucinations of circus clowns singing in her room and tormenting her to keep her awake. The surgeon would like to proceed with the procedure if she can give competent consent.

Since your first patient is not until 8:30 this morning, you decide to cut short your workout and see Ms. St. Laurent first thing this morning. Driving to the hospital, you take a call from Dr. White, an internist asking about a patient he is about to see this morning in his clinic. The patient, a "frequent-flier" in the hospital's emergency department, is a 45-year-old man who insists that something is "seriously wrong" with his heart and believes he has been having a series of "heart attacks." He has been in the emergency department four times in the past 3 weeks with shortness of breath, chest pain, lightheadedness, and intense fear. Typically, however, by the time the emergency room physician sees him, the worst of his symptoms have resolved. Despite two thorough cardiac evaluations (which were negative), the patient was not reassured and did not accept the strong probability that he was having panic attacks. At his last two emergency room visits, he has had an electrocardiogram and has been instructed to see your colleague for an office visit. He is finally appearing for an office visit – prompting the phone call. Dr. White adds that a representative from the patient's health insurance company has been calling the physician about the amount of cardiac testing that the patient has had. After indicating to Dr. White that you would be happy to see the patient later this week, you also suggest that he evaluate the patient further for possible panic disorder and remind Dr. White that selective serotonin reuptake inhibitor (SSRI) antidepressant medications are typically used to treat the condition.

7:55 a.m.

Ms. St. Laurent is indeed confused. When you ask her what season it is, she reminds you that "Christmas is just around the corner" even though it is mid-July. She cannot tell you why she is in the hospital and often responds to questions with incoherent rambling. However, during your 30-minute assessment, she also has brief bouts of clarity and can repeat seven digits forward, and at one point anxiously says, "Something's just not right with me." You note in her chart that, at this point in time, her mental status is fluctuating to such an extent that, in your judgment, she cannot provide genuine informed consent for surgery. However, you also write that the history of a sudden onset of confusion, together with the fluctuating consciousness that she demonstrated during your interview, strongly suggests a diagnosis of delirium. In your note, you suggest that she be further evaluated for a cause for her confusion and note that these states are often triggered by systemic illness and/or medication interactions.

8:45 a.m.

Your first patient has been waiting 15 minutes. This is a 7-year-old boy who you hear before you actually see. He is in the waiting area with his mother, and as you open the door you are greeted with a boy jumping off a chair. You observe that he appears to have thrown most of the waiting room's magazines all over the floor. As you are talking with the mother and the boy in your office, there is a knock on the door. Dr. Overman, another physician in the practice, asks if you can see a patient who is in exam room 12. Dr. Overman describes the patient as a 30-year-old woman who suddenly broke into uncontrolled sobbing when he walked into the exam room. He states that she seems to "have some kind of stress" and adds, "You're better with this sort of thing than I am and besides, I'm already behind – I've got two other patients I need to see."

After spending 10 more minutes with the mother and child, providing some questionnaires for mother, father, and the boy's teacher to complete, as well as scheduling a follow-up appointment, you go to exam room 12. You find a slightly disheveled woman sitting on the exam table sobbing while the nurse tries to console her. Upon your arrival, the nurse leaves, saying to the patient, "I'm sure you will feel much better after talking with the doctor," as she nods in your direction. In between sobs, the patient says that she has been "going out of my mind." Last night, she explains, her husband of 5 years told her that he was in love with another woman, packed some clothes, and left: "I came to the doctor because I didn't know what to do with myself. I couldn't go to work like this."

After you make some empathic comments and seem to have established rapport, the patient calms down a little and indicates that she is most concerned about the impact that this will have on her 4-year-old son. You and the patient develop a plan – she will ask her mother to stay with her for the next several days, you suggest that the physician provide her with a work excuse, and encourage the patient to contact her two sisters as well as her group of friends and finally, to consult with an attorney. You caution her against taking any significant action on her marriage at this time but do schedule her back for an appointment in 3 days. After she has calmed down somewhat, you leave the room, find Dr. Overman, briefly summarize the patient's situation and your plan, and encourage him to write the work excuse.

11:00 a.m.

You meet with a 40-year-old male who is a three-pack-a-day smoker. He explains that after a benign nodule appeared on his next neck about 3 months ago, he has decided to quit smoking, "This time, for good." He is also a patient of Dr. Overman. Because of the quantity and duration of his cigarette use, Dr. Overman has suggested a trial of medication – buproprion – to assist with cessation. After learning that the patient had tried cessation before but had only been able to go without smoking for less than 12 hours, you conclude that nicotine replacement is also likely to be helpful. Before you begin discussing environmental and behavioral smoking cessation strategies with the patient, you query him about symptoms of major depressive disorder. He seems to have at least five of the required symptoms for a Diagnostic and Statistical Manual of Mental Disorders (DSM) diagnosis of major depressive disorder. Recognizing that untreated depression will make cessation much more difficult, you suggest that the mood disorder be addressed first and that the smoking cessation protocol be initiated after those symptoms have improved. You step out of the room, find Dr. Overman, and briefly explain the situation. The physician responds: "Don't you think that if we can get him to stop smoking his depression will get better?" You explain the much poorer success rate for smoking cessation among depressed smokers and suggest that maybe the patient will be more likely to be successful in about 6 weeks, if the depression is promptly treated. Dr. Overman sighs, "Ok, you win," and pulls out his prescription pad: "What should I write for?" Since the patient had not been treated for depression previously, you tell the physician that as a general rule, any of the SSRIs would probably work equally well. Dr. Overman presses you: "Just tell me which one?" After pointing out that sertraline may have fewer side effects and a better record of adherence, he writes the script and hands it to you: "Tell him to schedule back with me in 2 weeks."

11:45 a.m.

You are now a half hour behind schedule. The pediatrician across the hall from your office has referred a 12-year-old boy to you who weighs approximately 180 pounds. His blood pressure is elevated. On entering the exam room, you are struck by the boy's size – he is bigger than you are. When you ask the patient and his mother about their understanding of their meeting with you, she immediately and firmly states that she does NOT believe that her son has any "psychological problems," just "slow metabolism." You do your best to diplomatically explain the risks of obesity, particularly in children, and recommend that the boy begin some type of regular physical activity – even if only walking 5–10 minutes a day as a start. You also refer the patient and his mother to a nutritionist at the local pediatric hospital. You write all this information down and give one copy of your recommendations to the boy and one to his mother, but you have a sinking feeling that they will not follow through. As they leave the office, you smell Chinese food.

12:30 p.m.

You go to the office conference area where a pharmaceutical representative is giving a luncheon. After getting some food and admiring the drug representative's Brooks Brothers' suit, you listen as he explains the benefits of a new medication for type II diabetes. Given the number of patients that you see regularly with this condition or who are at risk for type II diabetes, you listen, take some of the literature, and eat quickly.

12:45 p.m.

While you are eating, Dr. Smithson, another physician in the practice, asks if you will be around this afternoon. She explains that she has an elderly patient who is coming in with his daughter to see her. The daughter called Dr. Smithson expressing concern about her father continuing to live alone. He apparently has been forgetting to take his medication and does not seem to be bathing regularly. The daughter had recently arrived at her father's home to find the oven on, no food in the oven, and her father asleep on the sofa. You had hoped to get the morning's chart notes done early this afternoon, but it looks like they will have to wait until early evening.

1:15 p.m.

On your way back to your office area, you pick up two phone messages and several insurance company forms to complete. Before getting to your office, you are stopped by the office manager. She asks if she can talk to you for "just a second." She is concerned about the office receptionist who has been coming in progressively later in the morning for the past 2–3 weeks. The office manager adds, "Twice, I think I smelled alcohol on her breath. She is a good employee and I really don't want to fire her. Could you possibly see her?" This one sounds complicated and you think twice before answering. Given office politics, you know that there are likely to be other issues here but you have no idea what they are – only that you would like to avoid stepping on an office land mine. After a pause, you say, "Let me think about the situation and then I'd like to talk to you some more about it, maybe tomorrow when we both have some time." The office manager is not going to let you slide out of this one: "Okay then. Let's meet at 7:45 tomorrow morning before the patients start coming in."

1:45 p.m.

After taking a phone call and reviewing some records, you note that you are only 15 minutes behind schedule. The first patient of the afternoon is a 16-year-old girl who was recently seen by one of the family physicians in your group. The girl, Susan, is accompanied by her mother. The record indicates that Susan recently had episodes of fainting at school. Laboratory work suggested electrolyte imbalances. The family physician, fairly knowledgeable about mental health issues, asked Susan about her eating habits as well as binging and purging behavior. Susan described episodes of purging three times a week as well as laxative use. While Susan appears to be of normal weight, her mother says that Susan is obsessed with her body image: "She asked if she could have liposuction for her birthday." Susan looks acutely embarrassed. You decide to ask a few more questions with the mother present and then to talk with Susan alone. After spending approximately 45 minutes with Susan and her mother, a fairly long time in your practice, you recommend a local intensive day treatment program for teenagers with eating disorders. After describing the program to the mother and daughter, they reluctantly agree to consider it.

2:45 p.m.

Dr. Smithson's 70-year-old patient and his daughter are in an examination room finishing up with the physician. While looking through his chart, your cell phone goes off. Apparently the teenage girl with eating disorder symptoms does not have a health insurance plan accepted by the treatment center. You speak briefly with the girl's mother, indicate that you will look into some alternatives, and contact her later today or early tomorrow. You also ask the name of the health insurance company and make a note to check with them about eating disorder treatments that they will authorize.

Dr. Smithson comes out of the examination room shaking her head. She says, "I'm really worried about having this guy live alone much longer. Let me know what you think." After introducing yourself to the patient and his daughter, you ask the patient if he understands why he is here. He says, "To get a checkup." You go on and ask him directly if he has noted any changes in his thinking, attention, or memory. He says, "I'm just fine. I don't know what all this fuss is about" and glares at his daughter. You feel the tension in the room and decide that it might be better to briefly separate the two. You ask the patient and his daughter if it would be okay if you saw the patient alone and then, looking directly at the patient, ask if it would be okay if you spoke with his daughter by herself as well. You explain that oftentimes it is difficult to talk about family members in front of them because adult children do not want to hurt their parents' feelings. He is agreeable to this and you spend the next 45 minutes assessing the patient with the Mini-Mental Status Examination (MMSE), screening for depression, inquiring about medications and alcohol use, and then speaking with the daughter, alone. The patient does demonstrate some mild difficulties with short-term memory that do appear to be slightly greater than would be expected for his age. Moreover, the daughter does appear to be extremely worried about her father's safety. You close the visit by indicating that you would like to see the father again in several weeks, repeat the MMSE to help determine if the memory changes you detected are transient or stable, as well as speak with the physician about how she would like to manage the patient's living situation. For the interim, you ask the patient if he would mind if his daughter checked on him on a daily basis, and tell the daughter that if there is anything that is concerning to her that she can contact you or Dr. Smithson. The father agrees to this plan and the daughter appears relieved.

4:00 p.m.

After gathering up some notes and presentation materials, you head over to the nearby university where you are teaching in the graduate program in psychology. As soon as you pull into the parking lot, your cell phone goes off again. Dr. White's office is calling – the patient with the anxiety/cardiac symptoms who you and the physician had discussed early that morning just called the office and was very distressed. He took his first dose of fluoxetine several hours ago and says he is nauseous, the room is spinning, and he feels jumpy. You encourage the office staff to let Dr. White know and point out that the patient's reaction to beginning an SSRI is not uncommon and will typically get better in about 5 days.

You return to your class preparation. This semester you are teaching a course on theories of psychotherapy and personality. Today's topic is Jungian analysis. Sitting in your car in the university parking lot, as you glance through your notes reviewing concepts such as archetypes, the ego, and the integration of the self, you smile. This class, which is much like the one you took during your graduate training in clinical psychology, seems a world away from the type of psychology that you practice everyday.

Overview of the Book

This psychologist's workday is very different from the one for which most mental health professionals were trained. It is fast paced, full of surprises and interruptions, and includes a wide variety of clinical problems across the lifespan. Time is of the essence. "Running behind," with scheduled activities interrupted by patients and events requiring a rapid response, is a daily challenge. The uninterrupted 50-minute psychotherapy hour is rare. Regular challenges include determining when symptoms are due to a mental health versus a nonpsychiatric medical condition as well as the ability to assess, diagnose, and make treatment decisions quickly. These determinations must be made without the benefit of the "full battery" of psychological tests that many psychologists were trained to see as the only way to do a "real" evaluation.

Philosophically, primary care physicians and mental health officials have had very different professional and educational socialization and, as a result, approach patients differently. Additionally, the two professions are trained to see patients in very different contexts. The traditional psychologist's private office with stuffed chairs, sofas, and artwork on the walls is a world away from the austere exam room and general hospital suite of the medical setting. While mental health problems occupy a good deal of the daily work of a pediatrician, family physician, or internist, their patients often present these symptoms very differently in primary care as opposed to the mental health setting. Primary care patients with psychiatric issues also differ from those seen in mental health settings, since symptoms of depression or anxiety are likely to be part of a clinical picture that includes hypertension, asthma, type II diabetes, or other physical problems.

The growing area of clinical health psychology has included useful techniques for addressing public health problems such as obesity, smoking, lack of physical activity, poor diet, and alcohol abuse. However, practicing psychologists often view these lifestyle risks as secondary to the diagnosis and treatment of psychiatric conditions as described in the Diagnostic and Statistical Manual (American Psychiatric Association, 2006). In primary care, however, and particularly with the growing prevalence of chronic illness in which lifestyle factors play an etiological role, these habits are among the most common presenting behavioral conditions.

Despite these realities, most psychologists, like the author, who have had rewarding careers in primary care, have been essentially self-trained. While postdoctoral psychology training programs in primary care are growing, and there is increased attention to collaboration between mental health and medical providers, there is still relatively little practical information to guide mental health clinicians new to this setting.

This book is designed as a practical guide for mental health professionals entering primary care, as well as for those who have had professional experience collaborating with primary care physicians. The book is divided into two major sections, the first basically about the primary care culture and the second primarily about interventions suited to this setting.

The first section, covering Chapters 1 through 4, describes the culture of primary care. It includes a description of the patients, their expectations, and common clinical problems. In many respects, patients in the primary care sector are more heterogeneous than those seen by most mental health professionals. It is generally assumed that when a patient appears in a psychotherapist's office, his or her chief concern is to address psychological distress. However, in primary care, the psychologist cannot make the same assumption. One of the major challenges in the general medical setting is "sorting out" symptoms and assigning them to diagnostic categories. Mental health professionals working in this setting will need to be aware that while symptoms of lethargy, insomnia, poor concentration, and lack of appetite characterize many mental health conditions, the same symptoms may signal a range of medical problems such as hyperthyroidism, hypothyroidism, cardiovascular disease, or type II diabetes, as well as interactions or side effects of medications used to treat medical conditions. Patients themselves interpret psychiatric symptoms as stemming from a physical condition and, understandably, see their medical doctor as the appropriate person to diagnose and treat their distress.

As the practice diary above suggests, the primary care setting is a unique culture with its own values, norms, language, and explanatory models. In my years of practicing, writing, and lecturing about primary care psychology, I always return to one implicit, yet critical principle: This culture will not be readily changed by even the most gifted mental health professional. I have seen many psychologists become frustrated and angry because the setting does not value their 15-page, single-spaced psychological evaluations, 13-generation genograms, or the year of weekly psychotherapy sessions that we have been trained to provide. Psychologists have much to offer their physician colleagues. However, efforts to change primary care practice so that it is more in line with psychologists' professional values are seriously misguided. Having an impact in this setting occurs when psychologists accept and work within the primary care culture and avoid the missionary zeal to transform their physician colleagues into "mini-psychotherapists."

Much of primary care work is consultation. While formal models of consultation (Caplan & Caplan, 1993) are familiar to most psychologists, consultation in primary care is often of the "curbside" variety: Physicians will stop you in the clinic corridor or contact you by phone when they have a spare minute to discuss patient issues. Reasons for consultation are sometimes obvious, but may also have a number of unspoken meanings. I owe a debt to the British National Health System, which has regularly employed counselors and therapists in general practitioners' offices for decades (Bor & McCann, 1999; Webster, 2002). These professionals have helped articulate many of the conflicts arising in primary care consultation that I have experienced but was unable to label (Bor & McCann, 1999). Finally, basic practice issues such as documentation, and ethical concerns such as dual relationships, will be explored in the early section of the book to provide an appropriate context for the latter section addressing specific psychotherapeutic interventions.

The first section concludes with a discussion of screening and applied epidemiology. A primary care practice cares for a small population of patients. As a result, epidemiological research, when applied thoughtfully, can assist with screening and diagnosis. Knowledge of risk factors for mental health conditions, as well as for behaviors such as smoking, excess alcohol use, and nonadherence, helps narrow the range of diagnostic possibilities in a heterogeneous patient population. Additionally, when intervention is viewed at a population level, brief counseling and screening have been demonstrated to reduce a population's alcohol use, smoking, and improve well-being. Because of the number of patients in an average primary care practice with psychiatric conditions or behavioral risk factors, psychologists, in order to have optimal impact, will need to implement brief and focused treatments.

The second section of the book focuses primarily upon brief interventions that either have been developed specifically for the primary care setting or have been adapted to this context. These approaches include targeted interventions for health risk behavior (the five A's; FRAMES), applications of the stages of change model to move patients toward healthier lifestyles, and motivational interviewing, a relatively new technique that emphasizes the role of patient values and personal investment in behavioral change. For larger-scale psychosocial issues, including relationship conflicts as well as mood and anxiety disorders, the BATHE technique and adaptations of narrative therapy will be useful. Patients who, like their physicians, are good logical problem solvers, will probably benefit from problem-solving oriented techniques. Acceptance and commitment therapy holds promise for increasing the coping skills of patients with chronic illness. Finally, the growing cultural diversity that influences patients' health behavior concludes the discussion of interventions.

Chapter 2

The Patients

When seeing patients in the primary care context, a useful distinction is that between disease and illness (Kleinman, 1988). Disease reflects the physician's perspective. This is usually a biological explanation reflecting some alteration in physiology and/or anatomy. Kleinman (1988) uses chest pain as an example. Chest pain is a fairly common presenting complaint. When chest pain can be diagnosed as treatable acute pneumonia, the disease model works well. Unfortunately, symptoms are usually not as directly linked to the disease state. Anginal-type chest pain, while reflecting coronary artery disease, may also reflect a long history of hypertension, discontinued pharmacotherapy because of erectile dysfunction and/or other side effects, family conflict, unrecognized anxiety, and the patient's own intense fear of death.

Illness, on the other hand, is the content of most day-to-day primary care practice. Illness describes "... how the sick person and the members of the family or wider social network perceive, live with, and respond to symptoms and disability" (Kleinman, 1988, p. 3). While many readers may consider upper respiratory symptoms to be the sine qua non of disease, most of the time these symptoms actually reflect illness. The majority of patients with upper respiratory symptoms do not have a clear bacterial cause leading to appropriate prescribing of antibiotics. However, both quantitative and qualitative studies have demonstrated that antibiotics are prescribed frequently when there is no evidence of bacterial cause. Why, then, do most patients who bring these symptoms to their physician receive a prescription for antibiotics? Qualitative studies indicate that there is an upper respiratory "dance" that occurs between physician and patient in which the patient uses several justifications for needing an antibiotic (fear of missing too much work, children missing school, prior positive experience with antibiotics, an emphasis on level of discomfort, and demanding "something" for it) (Scott et al., 2001), and physicians often respond with their opinion that the condition is viral and does not require an antibiotic. The dance may become more intense as the physician tells the patient about the growing concern about antibiotic-resistant infections that have developed – possibly from the inappropriate overuse of antibiotics. Still, more often than not, the patient leaves the office with a prescription.

What is happening here? While disease is present, the patient's illness experience becomes the central clinical issue. How did illness win out over disease – particularly when the physician has the prestige of biomedical research on their side? During the typical primary care encounter, patients bring illness complaints to the examination room that are translated into disease based upon a biomedical understanding of the complaints.

> Disease is what practitioners have been trained to see through the theoretical lenses ... [of their discipline] ... That is to say, the practitioner reconfigures the patient's and family's illness problems as narrow technical issues, disease problems (Kleinman, 1988, p. 5).

Sore throat, cough, runny nose, and stuffy head interfere with the patient's work and family life; it keeps the 8-year-old girl from her dance recital as well as from her second grade class; it contributes to further distancing between husband and wife in a marriage lacking in sex and affection. Successful primary care physicians are aware that they are dealing with illness and at times, may temporarily compromise the biomedical logic of disease in its favor.

Primary Care Patients *Are* Different

Patients seen by psychologists either referred by primary care physicians or seen in the primary care office differ significantly from those presenting in the traditional mental health sector. First, primary care patients do have high levels of psychiatric distress. However, psychiatric problems are rarely the problem bringing the patient to the physician's office. Second, primary care patients' mental health symptoms are intertwined with physical problems. At the same time, many of these physical complaints are vague and have no established etiology. While DSM-IV mental health conditions are common, primary care psychologists also spend a good deal of time dealing with a third problem type: behavioral issues that do not fall into a specific psychiatric category. These include obesity, diet, and sedentary activity, a desire to stop smoking, or difficulty adhering to a diabetic regimen. Furthermore, the patient's distress occurs within the context of developmental issues and life events including fears about being a good mother of a newborn, focused family crises such as the death of a child, divorce, job loss, or conflict with a work supervisor, and decisions about placement of aging relatives. Finally, physicians struggle with patients that have physical symptoms for which no etiology can be established. All of these challenges may coexist with ongoing chronic illness, such as type II diabetes or hypertension, acute problems such as the common cold or sinusitis, or health maintenance visits for regular physicals for work or school.

Demographics and Presenting Problems

Demographically, there appear to be differences between patients seeing primary care physicians for mental health problems versus those seeing a psychiatrist or psychologist in the mental health sector. Primary care patients with psychiatric conditions are likely to be male, older than age 65 years, and have less formal education. Additionally, primary care patients with mental health concerns are more likely to have comorbid substance abuse and medical conditions as well as being members of racial and ethnic minorities (Cwikel, Zilber, Feinson, & Lerner, 2008).

As noted above, patients with psychological/behavioral issues seen in the primary care setting are different in other ways than those seen in the specialty mental health sector. First, presenting problems are more likely to focus on physical distress rather than emotional or social difficulties. Second, primary care is also the setting for ongoing treatment of the growing number of patients with chronic illnesses such as asthma, hypertension, or type II diabetes. Finally, primary care is the major clinical context for routine medical visits such as school physicals as well as the setting for most preventive care.

Primary Care: The *De Facto* Mental Health System

Psychiatric symptoms are very common in primary care settings. In the United States, the primary care sector is the most common treatment setting for mental health problems (Cwikel et al., 2008). For example, 50% of all patients in the US treated for major depressive disorder are managed solely in the primary care sector. These physicians spend a total of 12.1 hours per week – nearly a quarter of their direct patient contact hours – providing mental health services. When directly compared on the basis of patient contact time, primary care providers see far more patients with mental health conditions than psychologists or professional counselors. Nationally, approximately 20% of psychotherapy sessions are provided by primary care physicians (Searight, 2007).

When compared with the general population, primary care patients have elevated levels of psychiatric symptoms. An early large-scale survey of primary care patients found that approximately 20% had a current psychiatric condition (Barrett, Barrett, Oxman, & Gerber, 1988) with major depressive and anxiety disorders being the most common. An additional 11% were diagnosed with another psychiatric condition. However, a number of these patients had comorbid depressive symptoms as well. Generalized anxiety disorder was the second most common mental health diagnosis. Of note, when examining the presence of symptoms rather than specific conditions, only 30% of this primary care population were free of psychiatric symptom with approximately 40% exhibiting mild symptoms (Barrett et al., 1988).

More recent studies suggest that rates of psychiatric distress in primary care are rising. When examining the prevalence of mental health conditions in primary care attendees during the past year, approximately half of all patients reported significant psychiatric symptoms (Cwikel et al., 2008). Women were more likely (54.8%) than men (44.9%) to be exhibiting significant psychiatric distress. When the more stringent criterion of meeting a formal DSM diagnosis was employed, 26% of men and 34% of women had a mood, anxiety, or eating disorder and/or somatoform disorder. While mood disorders were the most common with 17.4% of men and 22.2% of women meeting criteria for major depression during the past year, anxiety disorders were a close second with 13.5% of men and 20% of women having at least one of these disorders during the past year (Cwikel et al., 2008).

Among pediatric patients, the majority of diagnoses of attention deficit hyperactivity disorder are made by pediatricians and family physicians. When examined from the perspective of sheer numbers, the majority of prescriptions for stimulant medication used to treat the condition are also written by primary care physicians (Mayes, Bagwell, & Erkulwater, 2009).

Subsyndromal Psychiatric Conditions

Of particular note is the large percentage of patients with subthreshold psychiatric syndromes. Cwikel et al. (2008) found that approximately 15% of male and female primary care patients have at least some of the symptoms associated with cognitive impairment, depression, panic attack, or hypochondriasis. Other studies have found that these subthreshold psychiatric conditions are associated with high levels of impaired functioning and greater utilization of medical care.

Minor depression, similar to major depressive disorder (MDD) with the exception of requiring only 2–4 symptoms (rather than five) for 2 weeks to meet diagnostic criteria (Wagner et al., 2000), has been associated with similar levels of disability. Among a group of older primary care patients, subsyndromal depression was found to be persistent at 1 year follow-up and as in previous studies, predictive of poorer global functioning (Lyness, Chapman, McGriff, Drayer, & Duberstain, 2008). The construct of minor mood disorders was further supported by the finding that levels of impairment for minor depression were intermediate between a major depressive disorder group and those without mood disorder symptoms (Lyness et al., 2008). Minor depression also appears to have two longer-term outcomes of concern; the complement of minor symptoms may persist or develop into major depressive disorder over time (Lyness et al., 2008). While associated with significant disability, there is less consensus about treatment for minor, as compared with major, depressive disorder. Pharmacotherapies such as selective serotonin reuptake inhibitors and/or evidence-based psychotherapies of choice for MDD, such as cognitive behavioral and interpersonal therapy, may have some efficacy for minor mood disorder but benefits do not appear to be as pronounced.

While less frequently studied, subsyndromal anxiety symptoms also appear common and are associated with impaired functioning and poorer health status. In a large sample of Dutch women, approximately one third reported significant anxiety symptoms (Denollet, Maas, Knottnerus, Keyzer, & Pop, 2009). Symptoms, such as chronic worry, free-floating anxiety, and excessive fear or panic, were associated with increased mortality through atherosclerosis as well as cardiac death. Among a group of middle-aged women, subsyndromal anxiety symptoms, even when depression and other cardiac risk factors were controlled, were associated with increased rates of cardiovascular death. Of interest, anxiety symptoms also predicted later lung cancer death even when the effects of smoking were controlled (Denollet et al., 2009).

Finally, while not as thoroughly investigated, combined subsyndromal anxiety and depressive disorder is also associated with significant functional impairment. In this condition, patients do not meet formal diagnostic criteria for either a mood or anxiety disorder but have symptoms of both conditions (Roy-Byrne et al., 1994). Similar to the other "unofficial" psychiatric syndromes described above, this mixed condition is also associated with a greater number of physical symptoms, disability, and a greater likelihood of developing a major psychiatric disorder (Roy-Byrne et al., 1994). The absence of clear guidelines or research evidence to make treatment decisions is another similarity shared with subsyndromal depression.

Detection of Psychiatric Conditions in Primary Care

Survey estimates suggest that between 20% and 60% of primary care patients have undiagnosed mental health conditions. While these conditions are common in primary care, multiple studies indicate that physicians often fail to recognize and formally diagnose these conditions. Two decades of research have concluded that an average of only 20–30% of these patients are detected. However, since the presentation of psychiatric symptoms in a primary care clinic differs from that found in a psychiatric practice, it is difficult and probably unfair, to view these physicians as in some way, negligent. There are several reasons for this pattern. First, in contrast to patients seen in the specialty mental health sector, primary care patients in psychological distress are more likely to focus on physiological symptoms. Thus, the depressed patient is likely to report fatigue and insomnia rather than dysphoric mood and lack of pleasure in usual activities as their chief complaint. Second, depressive and anxiety symptoms may coexist with a newly or previously diagnosed medical condition. This factor is particularly challenging to the physician since psychiatric symptoms overlap with symptoms indicating a medical diagnosis. Panic disorder patients, for example, are probably more likely to initially appear in a general hospital emergency department rather than a psychologist's office. Patients with panic disorder are likely to focus on particularly frightening physical symptoms such as chest pain, shortness of breath, lightheadedness, and near-fainting experiences. While panic symptoms may mimic a cardiovascular condition, there is also considerable evidence that anxiety disorders are more common among patients with previously diagnosed hypertension and heart disease than among persons without cardiovascular disease. Finally, the presenting problem may mask an underlying psychiatric condition (see also p. 21). Thus, tension headache and lower back pain often coexist with major depressive disorder and some would argue that headache is an expression of major depressive disorder (Searight, 1999). However, while somatic expression of psychological distress is particularly common in specific cultural groups such as those from the Middle East, the physician is likely to consider a mental health condition only after the appropriate battery of medical tests have been run and result in negative findings.

Patients Prefer Primary Care Counseling

While many mental health providers may find it difficult to believe that physicians seeing 20–30 patients per day can have significant relationships with any of them, many people view their doctor as the professional to whom they are most likely to turn when experiencing distress – physically, emotionally, or interpersonally. Additionally, because people see their physician at times in their lives when they are particularly vulnerable, there are strong elements of trust, gratitude, and security associated with the relationship. In many cases, the same physician has cared for the patient for decades. Finally, key developmental transitions often include the physician – births, early infancy, beginning school, retirement, and death. Family physicians, in particular, because they often care for entire families, often have a unique vantage point on a patient's psychosocial world. Some research suggests that medical patients are not particularly open to visiting a psychotherapist and prefer their primary care physician as a source for counseling. While nearly 90% of depressed primary care patients desired counseling, only 11% wanted to be referred for psychotherapist. Instead, they wanted their primary care physician to provide psychological treatment (Brody, Khaliq, & Thompson, 1997; Ruddy, Borresen, & Gunn, 2008).

Obstacles to psychotherapy, particularly in today's health care system, also make it more likely that patients will bring psychological difficulties to primary care providers. Patients often report that they have difficulty accessing mental health services, are placed on extended waitlists, or that the only available psychotherapist is geographically distant or can only see the patient at inconvenient times. Additionally, rising patient copayments make specialty mental health care increasingly expensive. There is less stigma associated with seeing a primary care physician as opposed to a psychologist. Because of concerns about maintaining health and life insurance, there is often fear that this sensitive information would be disclosed to third parties (Ruddy et al., 2008). Navigating the carved out mental health system is often extremely challenging and discouraging and frequently is an obstacle to continuity of care. In addition, even when the physician does recommend a particular psychotherapist with whom they have a working relationship; patients may encounter significant managed-care barriers to seeing this provider. Finally, prior negative experiences with the mental health system will also make it more likely that patients will turn to their trusted physician when experiencing psychological distress.

The trust that patients place in their physician often has a "halo" effect that extends to consultants to whom they refer. Patients referred to mental health professionals often begin the visit with "I don't know exactly why I am seeing you but Dr. Reed recommended you and that's good enough for me." In this way, the primary care provider's "halo" can extend to psychologists. Physicians are far more comfortable referring their patients to someone they know, have shared previous patients with in the past, and with whom they periodically communicate. For patients who seem reluctant to act on a mental health referral, their physician's brief testimonial can make a significant difference. (I know that there are a lot of therapists who practice in the community – just look in the Yellow Pages. I prefer to refer to Dr. Huber – she is someone that I know and she's had very good results with many of my patients.) (Ruddy et al., 2008).

Who Wants Long-Term Psychotherapy?

For years, a debate in the psychotherapy outcome literature has centered on the definition of treatment dropout. Is treatment complete when the psychologist says it is or when the patient draws this conclusion? In mental health centers, dropout rates range from 30% to 60% while in so-called centers of excellence, dropout rates may be as low as 17% (Waskett, 1999). Carey and Mullan (2007) found that the median number of counseling sessions attended by patients who did follow up with a physician referral for mental health care was one. When patients were clearly informed that the length of treatment was up to them, the median number of sessions was also one. Globally, studies of counseling in primary care indicate that patients do exhibit significant reductions in self-reported depressive and anxiety symptoms with brief counseling. Of note, several studies have found that patients are usually very satisfied with their counseling and therapy experiences (Seligman, 1995).

As noted earlier, patients are often very attached to their primary care physician. Patients tend to see their physician during episodes of illness and/or regular checkups. When the illness episode has resolved, patients are unlikely to have contact until a need arises again. While research on this process is nonexistent, the author's 18 years of experience of seeing patients in a family medicine setting suggests that patients' contact with the primary care psychologist follows a similar pattern. Patients would see the psychologist for 2–3 visits and may not see the psychologist again for several years. At that time, either a new life stressor emerged or psychiatric symptoms returned and the patient was seen again. The patient's distress would lead to another episode of several treatment sessions until the patient regained equilibrium and then direct contact ceased. The availability of the primary care psychologist in their physician's office group also is, on its own, very reassuring to patients. Even when the psychologist's contact with a patient was simply a "hello" in the clinic corridor, patients seemed to experience a sense of security in knowing that the psychologist was still there.

With the national average of 3–4 psychotherapy sessions attended for those who initiate treatment with a mental health professional, one can conclude that patients have been telling us for many years that psychotherapy would be brief. These data may provide some reassurance to psychologists new to this setting who are concerned that limited treatment will lead to patient dissatisfaction.

Somatization: It Is More Than You Think

While psychologists certainly have their share of diagnostic challenges, one could argue that they are small compared to those that daily confront the primary care physician. While important, mental health is a small part of the primary care provider's clinical knowledge base. Fatigue, chest pain, insomnia, and cognitive difficulties are symptoms associated with a multitude of conditions ranging from myocardial infarction to hypothyroidism to traumatic brain injury to minor depression or an adjustment disorder. Most psychologists have some exposure to somatoform conditions. However, as presented in most overviews of psychiatric diagnosis, somatoform disorders tend to be equated with conversion symptoms. These are typically seen as being of historic interest and as dramatic oddities but as having little bearing on day-to-day practice.

However, somatization is a common process in primary care. When looking at the phenomenon from the broadest perspective, primary care physicians deal with various forms of somatization everyday. In a now classic study, Koroenke and Manglesdorf (1989) found that approximately 80% of the physical complaints that were brought to primary care physicians had no established cause. These investigators examined the top 14 complaints in primary care and also calculated the percentage of patients with each complaint in which it was possible to establish a definitive cause for the symptoms. These symptoms included lower back pain, fatigue, limb pain, headache, and respiratory symptoms among others. Of these complaints, only about 10% of the cases had a clear established cause. If the term "somatoform disorder" is used to refer to medical conditions in which an etiology cannot be established, primary care physicians spend the majority of their working day dealing with variations on somatization.

Several authors have suggested that somatoform conditions are on the increase in the United States. Survey data obtained within several months of the destruction of the World Trade Center in September 2001 found that there seemed to be an elevation in the number of nonspecific somatic complaints reported. One model suggested is that a heightened awareness of unpredictable attacks upon civilians in Western countries leads to increased levels of autonomic arousal, which, in turn, is often experienced as physical discomfort.

Another large-scale social factor likely contributing to the increase in somatization is the direct marketing of pharmaceuticals to the general public. Historically, advertising prescription medication was considered unprofessional and inappropriate. In the 1990s, this barrier fell and since that time, many medications for a range of difficulties from depression to hypercholesterolemia to chronic fatigue to hypertension and urinary incontinence are all advertised, often very dramatically, to consumers (Barsky & Borus, 1995; Conrad, 2007). There is growing evidence that physicians are experiencing an increase in the percentage of patients who come to them almost self-diagnosed and requesting a specific treatment.

A closely related factor is the availability of health and medical information on the Internet. Many individuals who experience a circumscribed complaint or a nonspecific symptom, such as fatigue, will respond by searching potential causes and treatments online. Similar to the pattern of pharmaceutical requests, patients increasingly are arriving at their physician's offices with printouts from the Internet. Many of these include self-report questionnaires in which patients reporting a certain number of symptoms are strongly recommended to see their physician. Among patients who have a number of nonspecific complaints, probability alone will often result in them meeting the threshold number of symptoms to trigger a physician office visit.

Characteristics of Patients Prone to Somatization

Research to date has suggested two personality styles associated with increased sensitivity to physical distress. The first style, somatosensory amplification, is an increased sensitivity to benign physical sensations. People who are high on this characteristic will report that they are acutely aware of things occurring in their body – they experience their pulse or heartbeat throbbing in their ears, are very sensitive to hot and cold, have low tolerance for pain, are sensitive to hunger contractions, and react strongly to very mild discomfort like an insect bite (Barsky & Borus, 1995).

The second personality style, alexythymia, a condition in which patients have difficulty recognizing and articulating mood states, has also been found to be associated with somatization. Alexythymia appears to be more common in men and is a state in which individuals are essentially cut off from their emotional life. While this personality predisposition may seem to be the polar opposite of somatosensory amplification, there are some similarities. Those with this trait are relatively insensitive to mood states but express these characteristics through physical sensations. This pattern, including the lack of psychological mindedness, is consistent with psychodynamic explanations of physical sensations as a "safe" focus for an expression of physical distress. For example, patients with alexythymia are more likely to focus upon the physical symptoms of major depressive disorder while minimizing sadness, irritability, or dysphoric mood. When asked by a clinician if they feel depressed, these patients are likely to respond with, "Well, I'm not eating. I am not sleeping. I can't concentrate and I have very little energy. Wouldn't you be depressed too?" If any emotional distress is recognized and reported, it is seen as secondary to physical symptoms. Several studies have found that patients who focus on the physical symptoms of depression actually function at a somewhat higher level than those with the diagnosis who emphasize abnormal mood and cognitive factors such as helplessness and hopelessness.

While the most common description of patients with nonspecific somatic complaints focuses on their lack of psychological mindedness to the extent that these patients angrily reject any suggestion that their physical symptoms may be related to psychological issues, more recent conceptualizations suggest that these patients may be more heterogeneous. While the personality styles of alexythymia and somatosensory amplification are probably the most common, patients do vary along a continuum in their recognition of the role of psychological factors in physical distress. Among primary care patients, there appear to be four basic types. First, there is a "psychosocial type" who readily volunteers that their physical symptoms are likely to be related to stress. For example, "I don't think it is any surprise that my headaches began on the day after I got fired from my job. I'll bet my job and getting fired caused these." A second group of patients initially have a narrow focus on somatic distress but if queried further about their lives and the possible relationship between their symptoms and life stressors will accept a psychosocial formulation. These patients may say, "Well, yeah, um, now that you mention it there may be some things going on at home that might be making my pain worse."

The third type, the facultative group, may accept a connection if it is explicitly made by the provider. For example, a clinician may say, "It says here in your record that your father died 3 months ago – do you think that the ringing in your ears might be in some way related to your loss?" Finally, are the classic somatizers who will become very angry and defensive if any attempts are made to link physical symptoms to psychosocial distress. These patients are the ones that tend to be most frustrating for physicians. They are costly in that they are high utilizers of all health care services including specialist visits and diagnostic tests. However, while their symptom presentation often involves vague and changing symptoms, these patients are very sensitive to any implication that psychological factors may play a role. Causes of classic somatoform disorder have been fairly well articulated. These patients are likely to be raised in families in which one or both parents are heavily focused on their own somatic sensations and are also high utilizers of health care services. This pattern is both modeled for children and fairly quickly, the children themselves, because of frequent parental questions about symptoms, become hyperattuned to any physical distress (Mullins & Olson, 1990; Searight, 1999). The most common childhood version of somatoform disorder is recurrent abdominal pain. The vast majority of children who have recurring abdominal pain (stomach aches) are not found to have any physiological factor accounting for their pain. Of interest, a significant portion of these children when followed over time will continue to have both abdominal pain but will also develop other nonspecific symptoms including headaches and rashes.

Physician's Views of Patients Expressing Psychological Distress Through Physical Symptoms

Patients, like those described above, particularly the fourth type, with vague complaints that will not accept a psychological explanation, are the source of considerable frustration among physicians. While most of the medical specialties have a proportion of these patients such as ear, nose, and throat specialists who see patients with nonspecific tinnitus or gastroenterologists seeing patients with abdominal pain and diarrhea with no specific cause or allergists whose patients appear to have a particularly pronounced response to generally benign stimuli such as new carpeting, the majority of these patients are seen by primary care physicians. One reason that they are particularly likely to be seen in the primary care sector is that their symptom picture often changes such that at one point in time they may have chiefly GI symptoms, later in the year, they have neurological symptoms such as tingling or lightheadedness, and still later, may develop nonspecific back pain.

Physicians are trained to be problem solvers and their professional socialization often leads them to regard patients with continuing symptoms as evidence of professional failure. Physicians will often describe a sinking sensation in the pit of their stomach when they see one of these frequent clinic attendees on their schedule for the day.

Reflecting medicine's frustration with these patients is a range of derogatory terms that have evolved to describe them. These include terms such as "psycho," "croc," and the acronym "GOMER standing for: Get Out of My Emergency Room."

Studies of how physicians respond to patients with unexplained symptoms suggest that there are a range of common strategies. It is important that psychologists have an awareness of these because they may be frequently contacted to deal with these patients. Primary care providers try to maintain a balance between specialist referrals and handling patients' complaints themselves. However, some physicians become aware that they are developing a mindset in which they do not take frequent presenters to their office with adequate seriousness. Some physicians indicated that the more symptoms the patient complained of, the less credible they were seen and the more likely that the physician was to demonstrate low levels of interest and energy in working with them (Ringsberg & Krantz, 2006). Primary care physicians also reported that, even after detailed investigations did not reveal any explanation for symptoms, patients had an experience of becoming "stuck." Physicians indicated that their experience was similar: "When you can't find the line to pursue when the patient's teeth chatter and his or her knees ache" (Ringsberg & Krantz, 2006, p. 112). Finally, physicians would "buy time" by providing "sick notes" for patients allowing time off from their job, documentation for disability compensation, or supporting early retirement.

Somatization Reconsidered

It has been argued that patients with multiple somatic complaints are actually cooperating with their physician. Mental health issues are not part of their list of presenting complaints. While freely reporting lower back pain, fatigue, headaches, chest pain, heart palpitations, insomnia, and GI distress, primary care patients are far less likely to describe dysphoric or anxious mood or difficult life circumstances as their primary reason for seeking health care. By presenting physical rather than psychosocial symptoms, patients speak the familiar language of medical practice – a language with protocols, differential diagnoses, laboratory tests, physical findings, and empirical treatments rather than the more ambiguous and complex world of psychological distress. Physicians are more comfortable working up chest pain rather than a childhood history of trauma, headache rather than martial conflict, and fatigue rather than job loss (Barsky & Borus, 1995; Epstein, Quill, & McWhiney, 1999).

In addition to "speaking the physician's language" physical complaints also avoid the stigma of mental illness (Epstein et al., 1999). In fact, medicine has evolved a range of diagnostic terms to provide labels for these patients' complaints so that they fall within a medical framework. Labels, such as recurrent abdominal pain, somatic dysfunction syndrome, and nonspecific musculoskeletal pain, are ways that physicians can recategorize psychosocial distress in a familiar biomedical language.

This medicalization is supported by both physician and patient. From the physician's perspective, somatic complaints typically have either explicit or implicit protocols for evaluation and treatment. From the patient's perspective, they are given a diagnosis in which there is a clear implication of their condition being organic and also one which leads to a particular set of medical recommendations for further assessment or treatment. However, more recent investigations have suggested that this relationship between "functional and organic" disease is perhaps illusory. While early research indicated that patients presenting with multiple physical complaints were increasingly likely to have a mood or anxiety disorder as the number of physical complaints increased, recent studies have suggested a more complicated relationship.

Mussell et al. (2008) found that when examining gastrointestinal (GI) symptoms, the number of symptoms was a predictor of the presence of comorbid depression and/or anxiety disorder. For example, as the number of GI symptoms increased from zero to three the likelihood of a comorbid panic disorder increased from 5% to almost 27%. Similar patterns of relationship were found for posttraumatic stress disorder, social anxiety disorder, and generalized anxiety disorder (Mussell et al., 2008). However, in this study and other recent explorations, it was surprisingly found that both medically explained and unexplained symptoms had similar associations with depression and generalized anxiety. For example, while patients with dyspepsia were more likely to report psychological distress than individuals in the general population, those with functional versus organic dyspepsia did not differ in terms of their number of psychiatric symptoms. Mussell et al. (2008) found similar patterns when examining other GI symptoms. While these newer data indicate that the physical complaints are more likely to be associated with psychological problems, particularly as the number of physical complaints increases, the distinction between functional and organic carries less meaning.

Unfortunately, the climate of litigation and the physician's own fear that they may have missed a significant medical problem often result in a number of repeated and costly medical tests. This is further complicated by the laws of probability – when a large number of laboratory tests are run, patients may have a positive finding by chance. This result, in turn, confirms for the patient that there is indeed something physically wrong.

The provider's conclusion that physical symptoms reflect psychiatric distress often occurs only after multiple medical tests rule out other possibilities. For example, conditions such as anemia and hypothyroidism often present as fatigue; anxiety may be related to hyperthyroidism, excess caffeine intake, or hypoglycemia (low blood sugar). It has been said that it takes a primary care physician a minimum of three office visits before they diagnose major depressive disorder in a new patient. While this may seem like an inordinate delay, it is important to remember that (1) patients do not typically focus on mental health symptoms; (2) an office visit's duration is approximately 13 minutes (Wedding & Mengel, 2004); and (3) more often than not, the patient does have some type of medical condition be it sinusitis, an allergic rash, or muscle sprain, at minimum.

In the initial encounter with a new patient referred to a psychologist after a medical work up has ruled out organic disease and the physician has suggested that the symptoms are likely to be due to a mental health condition, the psychologist should not assume that the patient necessarily agrees with the diagnosis. The patient, still, may not be convinced that there every biomedical stone has been left unturned. ("The doctor said this chest pain I've been having is because of panic attacks – How he can be so sure that there's nothing wrong with my heart?") Asking the patient about their own views and hypotheses about their symptoms is a rapport-building place for the psychologist to begin the consultation.

But Remember: Even Hypochondriacs Die of Something

Primary care psychologists must have an appreciation of the role of medical factors and not "jump the gun" and automatically assume that patient complaints reflect psychiatric illness. Particularly if the patient is still undergoing medical evaluation while seeing the psychologist, mental health professionals should be very cautious in assuming that symptoms are due to mental health problems. Even if the psychologist is unsure, they will engender more respect from their physician colleagues by being aware of other, nonpsychiatric etiologies. Research on patients diagnosed with somatoform disorders has found that approximately 10–20% actually had an organic illness causing their symptoms (Mullins & Olson, 1990; Robinson & James, 2005).

Taylor (2007) presents some dramatic examples of medical conditions masquerading as psychiatric conditions. For example, the parents of a 7-year-old boy were concerned about a decline in the quality of his schoolwork as well as increased irritability and forgetfulness. He also reported headaches and joint pain and was demonstrating evidence of difficulties with coordination. He was initially diagnosed with attention deficit/hyperactivity disorder. When symptoms persisted, he underwent a more detailed neurological evaluation which indicated Lyme disease (Fallon, Kochevar, Gaito, & Nields, 1998). With the appropriate ongoing antibiotic treatment, symptoms were alleviated. In another example, a 10-year-old girl became increasingly nervous and was making unusual facial expressions. She became preoccupied with cleanliness and felt that there were germs around the house. Tests indicated that the girl was positive for group A beta-hemolytic streptococcus (Guerrero, 2003; Taylor, 2007).

Some years ago, the author saw a 45-year-old male referred by his internist for psychological assessment and possible psychotherapy. The patient reported decreased interest in his work and not feeling like his "usual self." There was a recent history of some marital difficulties. On testing, the patient exhibited an unusual pattern of cognitive functioning – he seemed to have circumscribed difficulty with concentration. As the appointment concluded, he said, as an afterthought: "I don't know if this means anything but I have been so cold – we have the furnace turned up at home but I still have to have a couple of blankets." This was reported to the referring physician with a recommendation for further neurological evaluation. While depression had been suspected by the referring physician as well as the patient's wife, further testing revealed a pituitary tumor.

The MINTS (Robinson & James, 2005) acronym is a useful mnemonic to use when evaluating a new patient. They remind the interviewer to consider **M**etabolic abnormalities (e.g., diabetes, uremia, and kidney disease), **I**nfections (e.g., HIV/AIDS, pneumonia, and viral infection), **N**eoplasts (e.g., cerebral, renal, or pancreatic tumors), **T**rauma (i.e., postconcussion syndrome), and p**S**ychological (after ruling out other causes; reconsider organic illness if symptoms do not improve with reasonable psychotherapy and/or pharmacotherapy) (Robinson & James, 2005).

Conclusion

Psychological practice in primary care involves attention to conditions and comorbidities that differ from the mental health sector. The coexistence of medical and psychiatric syndromes, subsyndromal variants of mood and anxiety disorders, as well as various forms of somatization present unique diagnostic and treatment challenges.

When evaluating a new patient, primary care psychologists should be vigilant to the possibility of medical conditions contributing to the patient's presentation. A strategy that the author has used in consulting on patients newly admitted to the hospital is to repeatedly ask himself if any aspects of the patients' symptoms and/or history are *inconsistent* with a psychiatric diagnosis. This may help with reducing diagnostic "blind spots."

Chapter 3

The Culture of Primary Care and Your Physician Colleagues

The Functions of Primary Medical Care

According to the Institute of Medicine's Commission on the Future of Primary Care (1994; Cassell, 1997), there are five basic assumptions about the role of primary care in the US health care system:

1. Primary care will be the logical foundation of an effective health care system because primary care can address a large majority of the health problems present in the general population.
2. Primary care will be essential to achieving objectives that together constitute value in health care, including quality of care, patient satisfaction, achievement of desired health outcomes, and efficient use of resources.
3. Personal interactions, including trusted partnerships between patients and clinicians, will be central to primary care.
4. Primary care will be an important instrument for achieving a greater emphasis on (a) health promotion and disease prevention and (b) the chronically ill – especially the elderly with multiple medical problems.
5. The trend toward integrated health care delivery systems will continue and provide both opportunities and challenges for primary care (Cassell, 1997).

In 2004, the *Future of Family Medicine Project* final report was published. This report was based upon a national survey of patients, payers, medical students, family physicians, and other clinicians. The report recognized that there had been initial optimism about primary care's development focusing on the centrality of primary care in a managed care system. However, the report also recognized that the promise of having a central medical "home" for patients had not been realized. The proposed model of family medicine contains the following elements:

1. Personal medical home: The primary care practice should be undertaken in a medical home for every patient including comprehensive integrated care in the context of an ongoing relationship.

2. Patient-centered care: A recognition that patients are active participants in managing their health and effective primary care practice featuring "... a patient centered relationship oriented culture that emphasizes the importance of meeting people's needs." (Future of Family Medicine Report, 2004).

3. A team approach: The recognition that health care is delivered through a system of professionals in multiple disciplines who provide ongoing care for a specific population.

4. Elimination of barriers to access: Innovations such as open scheduling, expanded office hours, and alternative forms of communication between patients and practice staff (such as e-mail) were encouraged.

5. Advanced information systems: Electronic medical records were described as the "central nervous system of the practice."

6. Redesigned offices: Offices should be practice centers that are designed to be responsive to patient needs and to ensure efficiency as well as comfort for both clinician and patient.

7. A whole person orientation: An emphasis on integrating care by the primary care practice rather than simply coordinating or organizing care.

8. Care provided within a community context: Health care should reflect a population perspective including cultural sensitivity to the specific population served.

9. Emphasis on quality and safety: A recognition of the need for ongoing total quality management and attention to factors associated with errors in patient care and reducing the influence of these errors.

10. Finances: Assistance in the development of new revenue streams that should contribute to greater financial viability of primary care practices.

11. Commitment to providing family medicine's "basket of services": A full array of medical services will be provided either directly or indirectly through established relationships with other clinicians.

As is evident from these descriptions, these systems of care include multiple roles for psychologists. The language of contemporary primary care focuses on integration, attention to patient-centered care, multidisciplinary teams, and culture. All of these dimensions are ones in which psychologists have significant expertise and can exert significant influence. While managed care was, in many respects, responsible for the rise of primary care, these health care generalists are likely to remain at the core of currently evolving health care practice models. At the time of this writing, the United States is once again considering some type of universal health care coverage. It is extremely likely that primary care would be at the center of any new health care system.

The Worldviews of Mental Health Professionals and Physicians

Primary care physicians and mental health professionals view the world through different lenses. These distinct perspectives are often the basis of confusion, disappointment, frustration and at times, even animosity, between primary care physicians and mental health professionals. Some common physician complaints about psychologists: "They spend nearly an hour with their patients and nothing seems to be accomplished; the patient doesn't get any better." "They spend week after week talking to patients about their childhood. There's no sense of urgency. This patient is gonna die if he doesn't quit smoking and drinking soon." Criticism is also leveled at psychologists because of the curtain of privacy that surrounds their work with patients: "You never know what happens to your patient when you send them to one of those people [mental health professionals]; it's like the patent has fallen into a black hole." Physicians often see psychologists as mired in reflection at the expense of meaningful, pragmatic action:

> They make things so complicated. I don't need to hear about the patient's extended family back to the Mayflower or his deep seated Oedipal conflicts. I just need to get this guy back to work.

Time is also seen very differently by primary care providers compared with mental health professionals:

> It took 3 months for my patient to get a psychiatrist's appointment – even though she was suicidal. First, I'm pleasantly surprised that she's still alive to go for the consultation. Second, after all that time waiting, the psychiatrist put her on Zoloft – I could've done that months ago.

Finally, physicians often find the professional communication of mental health professionals to be overly elaborated, delayed, and needlessly equivocal:

> I sent a patient to a psychologist for testing. Two months after the appointment, I got a 15 page report with pages of test scores and psychobabble. All I wanted to know was if my patient had Alzheimer's. I don't need a 50,000 word biography – Does the patient have Alzheimer's? *Yes or no.*

Psychologists have a different litany of criticisms for their medical colleagues. Physicians are often characterized as thoughtless pragmatists: "Those docs don't really help patients understand their problem or even try to get them to change their behavior. Their answer to everything is to just throw drugs at the patient." In addition, the high volume of patients, together with time constraints, contributes to a view that physicians are unreflective technicians: "They're so rushed, being a patient in their office is like being a car on an assembly line, next, next. ...."; "Those docs don't know their patients. They don't take the *time* to get to know them." Mental health professionals often cite their physician colleagues for their perceived lack of knowledge about psychological disorders: "They can't diagnose simple things like Attention Deficit Hyperactivity Disorder (AD/HD) or major depressive disorder unless it hits the doc over the head."; "Maybe they missed lectures the day that personality disorders were covered in med school – there *is* such a thing as chronic psychopathology." Even when they are given credit for their rudimentary knowledge base in behavioral science, mental health professionals fault physicians for their inability to appreciate the complexity of psychological treatment: "Those internists think I am going to cure a patient with borderline personality in a single visit?!" Those family doctors think that everything is straightforward and uncomplicated – when I try to explain that the patient is very complex, they get irritated with me and won't let me finish my description of the patient and interrupt with "Does she have panic disorder? Yes or no. Which meds should I start her on?" and their idea of empathy is to say, "I had a runny nose once, I got over it."

Many of these differences stem from distinct patterns of professional socialization, the settings in which clinical training and graduate education occur, and distinct pedagogical philosophies in medicine and psychology. Key differences include views of time, comfort with ambiguity, relative emphasis on pragmatism versus conceptual theorizing, communication (both with patients and professional colleagues), tolerance for irrationality and views of what constitutes a good outcome or cure. These distinct worldviews between physicians and psychologists are reflected in views of illness, expected and accepted treatments, as well as patterns of professional-patient interaction.

The Culture of the Primary Care Clinic

"You Can Observe a Lot by Just Watching." – Yogi Berra

For those completing conventional graduate training in psychology, entering a medical setting is like visiting a foreign country. The language differs (RBCs, neutrophils, MI, STAT, and LP), clothing (white coats), the sense of urgency, interacting with patients. (Mr. Ambrose – here is what you need to do; you need to lay off the beer and cigarettes for awhile.) The pace of events will seem like a whirlwind, conversations will begin but be interrupted by phone calls, a nurse's question or a laboratory report will be thrust into the physician's hand who glances at it and then disappears into an exam room.

For those new to the primary care setting, it is often helpful to ask a physician if you can "shadow" them for part of a day as they see patients in the clinic. Since this is often done by first and second year medical students, most physicians and patients are agreeable. If possible, it is extremely helpful to shadow different physicians and to observe on multiple occasions over time. The value in shadowing is that those new to primary care can obtain a much better understanding of how physicians work. It will also give the psychologist a much clearer picture of how behavioral and emotional issues are presented and addressed in this setting. As a clinical psychologist whose job it was to observe resident physicians and provide them with feedback about their patient interaction skills, I am certain I learned at least as much, if not more, from these experiences than the physicians I was training.

Primary care physicians are masters of efficiency. They are able to conduct a physical examination while maintaining an ongoing conversation about family or work stresses that the patient may be experiencing or assessing and counseling them about lifestyle change such as smoking cessation. While some traditionalists may wonder if patients are offended by this multitasking, observing primary care physicians at work will quickly dispel this notion. Actually, patients like to have some other topic to focus upon as a distraction from the poking and prodding that is taking place.

One of the best ways to understand the culture is to be an astute observer of the clinic – how nursing staff interact with patients, how physicians manage four patients simultaneously while reviewing laboratory results and X-rays of a patient that they saw earlier in the day, and their response to unscheduled patients or other surprises that occur during their clinic hours. Some other useful activities for psychologists are to attend medical conferences and grand rounds. Even if the content is not always comprehensible, observing the style, process, and organization of the presentation is helpful in developing an understanding of how physicians approach clinical problems. Medical conferences tend to be practical, rather than theoretical, and focus on differential diagnosis and/or treatment options. In contrast to psychology lectures, there is markedly less attention to etiology with more attention to the description of conditions, and accurate diagnosis which, in the presence of evidence-based guidelines for the problem, often leads directly to a therapeutic plan.

As we have suggested elsewhere, another useful source to better understand primary care culture is through its professional literature – particularly journals, such as American Family Physician, that are directed toward practicing physicians (Searight, Price, & Gafford, 2004). For mental health professionals, it is particularly educational to carefully review articles in these journals that address diagnosis and treatment of psychiatric problems in primary care. The nonmedically trained mental health professional will likely be struck by the emphasis placed on differentiating psychiatric from medical conditions and the reliance upon psychotropic medication as a treatment choice in these publications. The format of these articles also reveals a good deal about how primary care physicians reason and approach problems. Articles for practicing physicians are brief, concise, and include a number of subheadings and highlighted text in the margins to keep the reader on track. The number of tables and figures, particularly those with clinical algorithms, mnemonics (SIGECAPS – an acronym for remembering the symptoms of depression: S – sleep disturbance; I – interest reduced; G – guilt and self-blame, E – energy level; C – concentration problems; A – appetite/weight changes; P – psychomotor changes; and S – suicidal thoughts), stepwise protocols (e.g., A Systematic Approach to Evaluating the Patient with Abdominal Pain), and checklists (Six Things to Consider When Evaluating Memory Loss), is also noteworthy. Similar to primary care conferences, issues such as etiology receive far less journal space than differential diagnosis, guidelines for evaluation, and evidence-based treatments of choice. Even when addressing ambiguous physical signs or symptoms having multiple simultaneous causes, there is a clear preference for dualistic reasoning in which alternatives are eliminated (rule out myocardial infarction). While psychologists are often drawn toward making the simple more complex, medicine tends toward a reverse process of reductionism. This approach to clinical problems is important for psychologists to appreciate – particularly when communicating with physicians. Rather than an extended account of a patient's history and diagnostic possibilities, physicians will want "the bottom line."

Clinical Reasoning: Pragmatism Amid Ambiguity

While psychologists often take considerable professional pride in their ability to provide detailed, nuanced, descriptions of cognitive-emotional and personality processes, these skills are not as relevant in the primary care setting. Instead, this setting emphasizes the value of practical information that is immediately implementable and consequential for patient care (Searight et al., 2004). Rather than a detailed explanation of etiological theories of panic disorder, physicians will be much more interested in realistic, immediate treatment options such as selective serotonin reuptake inhibitor (SSRI) medications.

However, as noted in Chapter 2, these clinical decisions often occur in the context of a confusing array of patient reported symptoms. While many psychologists think of medicine as being objective and certain, in reality, ambiguity, and uncertainty abound – particularly in primary care. Most of the primary care physician's working day is spent addressing self-limiting illnesses that do not threaten life or bodily integrity. The positivist modern science in which physicians are trained often proves to be a very frustrating lens through which to view the array of patients that they see in an average clinic day. As Goldstein (1990) notes, the goal of the primary care physician is to make some sense out of the web of reported physical sensations and accompanying emotional and social meaning:

> I will insist on organizing ... [the patient's] ... feelings and the symptoms, fearlessly ignoring the symptoms that don't appear to contribute to the diagnosis ... first we filter the witnesses' reports in search of an interpretable pattern. We then apply a critical method of analysis to determine the reliability and validity of the information. I know from my unwary past that the patient will ignore the significant, exaggerate the trivial, and sometimes falsify the critical. I absorb everything the patient offers, transforming it from the idiosyncratic into knowledge with clinical meaning. The construction of therapeutic knowledge has begun (Goldstein, 1990, p. 5).

Goldstein notes that today's primary care physician must also appreciate the role of informal Internet consultants whom patients rely upon to aid in the interpretation of their symptoms:

> Daily, I discuss with patients the looseness of the semiotic connection between symptom and dread disease. Contrary to the American Cancer Society, "the seven warning signs of cancer" might be better classified as the "seven signs that could possibly mean cancer but probably only mean that you will be unnecessarily frightened and you will go through several unpleasant tasks before you are given back the peace of mind that it lost when you took the seven warning signs too seriously."

The worried well will always have a backdrop of symptoms that nearly all of us experience in an average 10-day period including itchy eyes, fatigue, headache, and muscle and joint pain (Barsky & Borus, 1995). For these patients, the availability of multiple sources of medical information at the click of a mouse can only make those benign symptoms seem more serious:

> My patients routinely terrify themselves by browsing through home medical encyclopedias until they find a diagnosis with a single match of symptoms. But until a symptom or sign is placed in the context of a patient's life, and the other symptoms or signs that the patient has or does not have, it is devoid of meaning (Goldstein, 1990, p. 5).

While Goldstein's account covers much of a primary care physician's typical office day, there is always the lurking threat of missing something more serious. While uncommon, the headache that reflects a developing brain tumor or the abdominal pain that is a sign of a cancerous tumor is always a dreaded possibility. Patients, their families, and importantly, their physicians, can be devastated by a missed diagnosis. This factor is a constant undercurrent in primary care medicine.

Even in the face of benign symptoms that will likely resolve on their own, most physicians still feel, and many patients expect, that the doctor should do something. This tension explains the large number of antibiotic prescriptions that are written for viral illness when the "textbook" treatment is rest and fluids. The pressure to treat these symptoms is nearly always present even when the correct diagnosis may not yet be known.

Physician education values emotional strength, quick thinking, and self-reliance. During medical school and residency, many physicians in training are routinely "pimped" by teaching physicians. Historically, the rapid-fire harsh questioning has been known to continue until the student breaks down in tears, is publicly humiliated, or both (Searight, 2007). The educational system also values endurance – an expectation that residents will provide round-the-clock patient care for 48 hours at a time. Recently, work hour restrictions were established for medical residents. However even these "reduced" hours are fairly draconian – no more than 80 hours per week with "only" 30 consecutive work hours. Even though research has found evidence for increased medical mistakes associated with sleep deprivation including a well-publicized study indicating that a residency work schedule may be associated with cognitive impairment comparable in magnitude to moderate alcohol ingestion (Arendt, Owens, Crouch, Stahl, & Carksdon, 2005), opposition to changing the system remains. Opponents of these more "humane" hours protest with the claim that staying up for several days at a time allows trainees to provide continuous patient care in hospitals and builds "character" in young physicians.

This tough, action-oriented, stance is often accompanied by a profound sense of responsibility. General descriptions of the personality traits associated with individuals in any profession will be flawed. However, medicine does place a strong value on traits such as perfectionism, conscientiousness, and responsibility (Myers & Gabbard, 2008; Searight, 2007). For psychologists who have the experience of being with medical residents responsible for overnight care in a hospital unit, they will note that even though a patient's death may be inevitable, there is a great sense of relief the next morning when the resident hands over responsibility for the patient to one of their peers. At least during this night, the patient did not die "on their watch." An understanding of this background may be helpful to psychologists who may be puzzled by their physician colleagues' periodic impatience and need to act.

This impatience, while not as intense, is often evident in dealing with patients whose compliance cannot be addressed through customary, rational, problem-solving strategies. As noted in Chapter 2, patients with a roving pattern of somatic complaints are particularly frustrating for physicians who may feel that they have somehow failed in correctly diagnosing a problem. The pragmatic, action-oriented approach that takes over oftentimes includes running more tests, referring patients to specialists, and providing written documentation of a disability to the patient's employer.

While many physicians in primary care are attuned to patient's psychosocial issues, there is still a propensity to address problems biomedically. The frequent appearance of antidepressant medications on the top 15 drugs prescribed in the United States attests to this value. Pharmaceutical companies have become well aware that most antidepressant prescriptions are written by primary care providers. In the past decade, these companies have directed their marketing and educational activities to this audience. They have made psychoactive drugs more accessible to primary care physicians by developing brief patient self-report measures to be used in primary care offices, emphasizing the safety and tolerability of medication, and stressing how widespread mental health problems are in this setting. While psychiatric education can certainly benefit primary care physicians, it does carry with it the implicit, if not explicit, message that psychiatric symptoms reflect physio-chemical conditions which are logically treated with medication – an approach with which physicians are comfortable.

Time

Time is probably the principal motivating and constraining force in medicine. Physicians are hyperaware of the passage of time. Efficiency is one of the most pervasive values influencing modern medicine. Psychologists typically do not have the same level of time consciousness as their medical colleagues. Much of this probably stems back to the history of the profession. The influence of training in long-term psychotherapy and the full battery of tests persist. Significant patient improvement occurring in on 1–2 sessions is a suspicious flight into health that does not reflect genuine enduring personality change or "cure."

Time has a very different economic meaning for primary care physicians as compared with customarily trained mental health professionals. Psychologists still often bill for services in terms of 50-minute intervals. However, while psychologists may complain about being scheduled tightly – these time frames are seen as luxuries by our primary care colleagues who are under pressure to keep office visits to 10–12 minutes – particularly in practices where productivity demands are high.

Physicians are consummate multitaskers. They are often looking to squeeze more activity out of every minute. Whenever any new practice technique or recordkeeping approach is suggested, the first thing physicians ask is "How much time does it take?" This question, usually asked with a suspicious tone, stems from the growing time crunch that governs medical practice. Similarly, whenever discussion of mental health problems includes suggested counseling techniques that physicians can use in their offices, an almost immediate response is "that will take too much time."

The average primary care visit is approximately 13 minutes (Gilchrist, Stange, Flocke, McCord, & Bourguet, 2004). In this time, the physician will address an average of three problems. In many primary care offices, it is not unusual for patients to be scheduled in 10-minute intervals. A specialist such as an orthopedist, who sees the patient after a nurse has interviewed and obtained X-rays, may spend less than 5 minutes in direct patient interaction.

One of the chief problems in teaching effective interviewing is that physicians tend to prevent patients from describing all of their complaints at the beginning of the visit. One classic study found that the average internist interrupted patients after they had only been speaking approximately 18 seconds in describing their presenting problem (Beckman & Frankel, 1984). While the time elapsed may seem agonizingly long to many physicians, researchers have found that the average patient completes their response to the question "what brings you in today" in under 60 seconds with nearly 90% of all patients completing their presenting problem description in under 2 minutes (Lipkin, Putnam, & Lazare, 1995). In Miller's (1992) study of the culture of primary care, seasoned physicians automatically scanned their clinic schedule each day looking for patients who would consume great deals of time versus those that that they could take care of very quickly. One of the chief obstacles to an efficient clinic session was difficult, multiproblem patients known as "schedule busters."

Psychologists new to the primary care setting may attempt to encourage physicians to use psychotherapy techniques with their patients. While many physicians are interested in psychotherapy and would like to implement these techniques, they do not see it is realistic. It is extremely important that psychologists appreciate that primary care physicians already feel an incredible time crunch – particularly when including the insurance forms and other paperwork that they must complete – and are typically not open to becoming "mini-psychotherapists."

Accessibility and Interruptions

In many mental health settings, the traditional uninterrupted 50-minute session is sacrosanct. Interruptions are rare and only for extreme events such as a fire in the waiting room. The cocoon of privacy that is the traditional therapist's office is temporarily insulated from outside activities including phone calls, pagers beeping, or knocks on the door.

If given the opportunity to shadow a physician during part of their office day, it will soon be apparent that interruptions are the norm rather than a rare exception. Pagers and cell phones erupt with frequency, nurses and physician colleagues knock on the door while Dr. Johnson is performing a rectal exam on Mr. Adams, medical assistants are summoned to the room to perform an electrocardiogram, and patients are directed out of the exam room with plastic cups in hand for urine samples. Successful physicians develop the ability to respond to these intrusions and to quickly return their attention to the patient.

To be successful in a primary care practice, psychologists should cultivate the same skill set. Extended uninterrupted visits are rare and the knock on the door or the phone ringing should be expected. A good way for a psychologist to quickly distance themselves from their primary care colleagues is to put a "Do Not Disturb" sign on their door when seeing patients. Over time, the ability to triage multiple patient and consultation demands becomes second nature. Mrs. Shapiro can complete a pencil-and-paper depression screen while the psychologist steps out to consult with a physician about a suicidal patient in exam room 7. While waiting for a physician to provide prescription antidepressant medication for the patient in your office, the psychologist may temporarily commandeer an exam room to begin smoking cessation counseling with another patient. Psychologists who are able to "dance" from patient to physician and onto another patient recognize this part of primary care culture. Unless the psychologist adapts their clinical style to the realities of the clinic, their impact on patients and value to their physician colleagues will be markedly reduced.

As was evident in the example in Chapter 1, this time pressure is even greater in general medical hospitals. Lengths of stay in these facilities are generally very brief. As soon as the patient is admitted, the focus immediately shifts to what needs to be done so they can be discharged. However, patients are often receiving multiple tests and procedures. Robinson and Baker (2006) note that it is not unusual for a patient to be in the hospital for 48 hours or less. The patient may be admitted late in the afternoon and needs to be seen by 3–5 practitioners prior to surgery which is scheduled for early the next morning. A consultation with the psychologist is requested at the time the patient comes to the hospital floor. The psychologist may need to come in later in the evening or very early the next morning to see the patient. The window of available time is often very brief and this limited time period is shared with other health care professionals (Robinson & Baker, 2006).

The Primary Care Psychologist's Approach to Patient Care

The Role of the Consultant

When physicians refer patients, there are varying levels of expectation about how active psychologists will be in the patient's care. In some instances, the physician, having exhausted their repertoire of medical assessment and intervention, will desire that the psychologist take over care of the patient. One clue to this expectation is when a patient is referred to a psychologist in the absence of medical follow-up visits. Probably the most common expectation is that the patient will be seen by the psychologist, assessed, and recommendations will be made to the physician. The third approach is that the physician and psychologist will work collaboratively and see the patient over time. This third pattern does not necessarily mean that the psychologist will see the patient in extended, intensive psychotherapy but will continue to follow the patient intermittently – often seeing the patient at closely spaced appointments until much of the immediate distress has resolved.

While primary care physicians do recognize that psychologists function somewhat differently than cardiologists, orthopedists, or oncologists, some expectations are similar. A good way to get a "feel" for the consultant relationship that primary care physicians have with specialists is to review letters and consultation notes submitted by consulting physicians, physical therapists, or other allied health professionals on specific patients that are being seen for behavioral assessment. While legal and ethical guidelines prohibit reviewing records of patients when the psychologist is not involved in their regular care, many patients referred to the psychologist have seen other consultants. Communicating with referral sources will be discussed further at the end of this chapter.

Two Common Forms of Consultation

While dated, a useful model for the mental health consultation was developed by Gerald Caplan in the 1960s (Caplan & Caplan, 1993). Caplan describes four basic types of consultation in mental health. Two of these approaches are most relevant for medical consultation. The first, client-centered case consultation, is the most common in medical settings. Here, the psychologist will evaluate a patient referred by a physician and provide diagnostic, treatment, and other relevant recommendations (e.g., the necessity of placement in a nursing home, admission to a psychiatric hospital) back to the consultee. In Caplan's model, even if recommended treatment could be provided by the consultant such as brief psychotherapy, intervention would not be initiated without the consultee's explicit authorization. This point is less rigidly followed in medical settings. However, psychologists recognize that when functioning as consultants, they are giving their professional opinion to the patient's physician. The consultee is responsible for the patient – not the consultant. The referring physician may follow the psychologist's recommendations or completely reject their advice.

In the second consultation model, consultee centered, the psychologist would not typically see the patient directly. The focus is on the consultee's (physician's) difficulty with the patient. In primary care, this is often through a "curbside" consultation in which the physician asks the psychologist for their advice on managing a patient in their practice. In this approach, the psychologist typically would not see the patient directly but would rely solely on the consultee's description as the basis for recommendations.

In this second approach, Caplan assumed that the consultee was experiencing psychological conflicts – largely unconscious – elicited by the case. These issues prevented the consultant from seeing the patient objectively and as a result, they could not accurately assess or treat the patient. While Caplan's psychodynamic formulation may be questioned, psychologists should be aware that patient referrals often reflect unspoken physician agendas.

Referrals

The Agenda Behind the Referral (Sometimes a Cigar Is Just a Cigar but Many Times It Is Not)

Referrals often reveal as much, if not more, about the referring physician than the patient. While many referrals are for focused issues (e.g., "Parent says she thinks child has AD/HD – please evaluate." or "65-year-old male with memory complaints. Assess mental status and report results."), other requests are not so clearly stated. Referral patterns also vary considerably with some physicians referring nearly all of their patients with mental health issues and others never making a referral or only sending very complicated patients. (Mr. Smith is a 47-year-old male with a 25 year history of alcohol dependence and schizophrenia who attempted suicide last week.)

Vague Referral Questions

While patients have underlying, unspoken agendas for the office visit, primary care physicians often have unarticulated reasons for referring patients to psychologists. These referrals, particularly when initiated by physicians with little prior exposure to psychologists as colleagues, often reflect a combination of patient management frustration as well as the physician's often unrecognized conflicts regarding responsibility, competence, and dependence. When the referral question is vague (social problems), dismissive (chronically noncompliant) administrative (Five sick notes in the past 2 months for back pain), or nearly absent (I just think he needs to see someone), the psychologist should respond with reflective curiosity and approach the patient and physician with supportive openness. For example, the patient requesting frequent sick notes often reflects a moral quandary for the physician that becomes more intense with each successive note written. The "sick note" patient may be referred because of either the physician's frustration with the patient and/or concern about the validity of the patient's repeated requests. Physicians recognize the need for supportive documentation for the "sick note" but at the same time are understandably uncomfortable with vague reasons such as "stress" as the rationale for work releases.

Inappropriate Referrals

For primary care physicians with little prior exposure to psychologists, the behavioral consultant may become a "dumping ground" for particularly difficult patients or viewed as a "resource" for patients with multiple social problems such as homelessness, poverty, lack of health insurance, or nonadherence with medical advice. While nonadherence may stem from depression or other psychological issues, frustrated physicians may also refer patients whose nonadherence stems from an inability to pay for prescription medication.

Another common type of referral is patients described as "draining." These patients, described in Chapter 2, often have multiple presenting problems, continue to bring up new complaints throughout the course of their office visit and from the physician's perspective, are "schedule busters" (Miller, 1992).

Referrals Representing Interprofessional Conflict

On a few occasions, the hidden agenda behind the referral may be professional struggles between two consultants or between a primary care physician and a consultant. In medical education programs, the psychologist may find themselves triangulated between an attending physician and a resident. Coupled with a strong sense of responsibility and perfectionism, correct diagnosis, and management is often a source of professional pride as well as personal self-worth. When a physician's judgment is challenged, or even mildly questioned by another physician, even if they are still in training, the specter of competence is instantly raised.

A clue to the possibility of a professional conflict is when the referring physician seems to be encouraging the psychologist to validate their assessment of a patient. ("I'm pretty sure Mr. Johnson is depressed, I just need for you to say so I can go ahead and treat him"). A tone of urgency associated with a referral for a nonlife-threatening condition is another clue that an interpersonal agenda may be present. (Physician: "Can you see this hyperactive kid *right away*?" Psychologist: "Is he a danger to someone? Did he get kicked out of school?" Physician: "No, but you really need to see him right away. Do you have any time today?") Rather than being reactive to the urgency, the physician's tone should be a clue to the psychologist to ask further about the situation. ("This referral sounds really important. Is there something else that would be helpful for me to know?").

Responding to Referrals

A psychologist who engages in reflective practice and who is able to use consultation and referral requests as an opportunity to collegially educate physicians about their role will be more likely to succeed as a primary care consultant. Initially, for the psychologist to become established – particularly with physicians with little experience working with mental health professionals – they should accept all referrals. However, this does not mean that the psychologist will necessarily treat or follow these patients over time.

Rather than simply being frustrated and resentful about inappropriate referrals, it is more valuable for the psychologist to "step back" from the referral question and conduct an independent assessment. Diagnosing and initiating treatment for a previously undetected psychiatric condition or attempting to learn from the patient's perspective, the factors that are contributing to their nonadherence with a diabetic regimen or repeated emergency department presentations for nonurgent reasons, can be helpful to both the consultee and the patient.

While being willing to see any patient at least once is a good policy for psychologists, it is the author's experience that to practice successfully in a primary care setting, it is necessary to set limits on the types of services provided. Many psychologists have been trained in conducting detailed psychoeducational evaluations for learning disabilities, child custody assessments in cases of divorce, preemployment evaluations for occupations such as police work, group therapy for sexual abuse victims, or extended marital and/or family therapy. While these are certainly important services, they can quickly fill the primary care psychologist's schedule leaving no time for new patients who should be seen quickly. Patients or their physicians, on learning of a psychologist's availability, may schedule an appointment expecting regular weekly long-term psychotherapy. Educating physicians by emphasizing your desire to be responsive to their consultation requests, having a good network of trusted mental health professionals to whom you can refer patients, and gently informing new patients of your practice pattern, should satisfactorily address these concerns.

At the beginning of a new patient visit with the psychologist, it is important that the patient be informed that the encounter will be problem focused. Framing your role as a consultant to the primary care physician and to the patient themselves will establish appropriate expectations at the outset.

When Should the Primary Care Psychologist Refer?

Over time, the primary care psychologist will likely develop a practice style similar to their physician colleagues. Patients will be followed over time with 1–3 visits when particular stressors arise. However, psychologists should have a network of colleagues who provide more traditional long-term therapy or specialized treatment (e.g., chemical dependency and eating disorders) as needed. Primary care physicians do understand the concept of specialty referral and with some explanation, are generally quite willing to accept this recommendation from the psychologist who supports their decision with a reasonable rationale.

Even if the referral issue cannot be realistically addressed in the primary care context, the psychologist who has a one-time consultation with the patient can provide useful information for the physician. For example, a 30-year-old woman with a 12-year history of three episodes a week of binging and purging is referred to you for "evaluation and treatment." In your judgment, the patient is unlikely to demonstrate much benefit from three to five sessions of primary care psychotherapy. However, the psychologist can provide a useful service by documenting the severity of the condition, previous treatment attempts, and recent history of physical problems or other psychiatric conditions. A primary care physician may not have had the time to obtain a thorough history of the patient's binging and purging, since this was not the patient's presenting problem, but will certainly appreciate having this information. When you describe the severity of the problem, as well as the previous treatment history and outcome, the primary care physician will certainly understand the need for specialized intensive treatment. In addition, if there is treatment that the physician could initiate while the patient waits for specialty care, this can be helpful as well. For example, in patients with eating disorders, rates of comorbid depression are very high and studies suggest that SSRI pharmacotherapy can reduce the frequency of binge eating. If there are no medical contraindications, the physician may initiate sertraline (Zoloft) and follow the patient at least until they could be seen in the specialty sector.

Finally, while most patients with psychological conditions can be managed collaboratively by a primary care physician and psychologist, there are a small percentage of patients warranting a psychiatric consultation. Consulting a psychiatrist should be considered with patients who are actively suicidal or psychotic. Depending upon the region of the country and population served, primary care physicians, while comfortable with mood and anxiety disorders, are often not comfortable treating bipolar illness or schizophrenic spectrum conditions. In some locales, a psychiatrist may see the patient once or twice a year with interim medication management by the primary care physician. Another situation in which a psychiatric consultation should be considered is when the primary care physician has tried at least two different trials of psychotropic medications for a mood or anxiety disorder and even though adherent, the patient has not demonstrated significant benefit. These treatment refractory patients are likely to require more than one psychotropic medication simultaneously – an approach with which many primary care physicians are uncomfortable.

Roles and Boundaries

Mental health education devotes considerable time to the importance of clear roles and professional boundaries. Ethical psychologists would never provide psychotherapy for family or friends. While we may have informal conversations with professional colleagues or office staff about personal and family matters, psychologists are discouraged from providing professional services to persons with whom they have another relationship – even if their sole contact is as a secretary or receptionist in their large group practice.

Primary care physicians, while being discouraged from treating friends and family, do not have the same degree of prohibition as psychologists regarding dual relationships. It is not uncommon for physicians to be the personal physician for office staff or even colleagues. While there are guidelines established by the American Medical Association for ethical practice, they are not as specific as the American Psychological Association's Ethical Principles in influencing practice or state licensing boards. In addition, the guidelines for nonpsychiatric physicians are not nearly as stringent regarding multiple relationships with patients.

Physicians who have not worked directly with a psychologist in the past may assume that the psychologist's perspective on personal and professional relationships is similar to their own. While treating family members is discouraged, it is not unusual for physicians to treat other physicians that they know, family members of colleagues, as well as employees of their hospital or clinic. The author's experience is that once the psychologist does become a valued member of a primary care practice, they often naturally will be viewed as *a*, and perhaps *the only* trusted, resource for psychological and interpersonal conflicts arising among the practice's physicians, nurses, and other office staff.

Mental health professionals, eager to be respected by their colleagues and coworkers, may feel considerable pressure to abrogate appropriate boundaries. It may initially enhance the psychologist's confidence to be sought out for counseling for personal matters by physicians and other medical staff. However, the primary care psychologist who does not heed their own discomfort about these conversations will soon understand experientially the rationale for APA's ethical guidelines regarding dual relationships. Psychologists should reflect upon and develop a policy for addressing these issues. For example, a member of the office staff may wish to talk with you about their difficulty in handling the death of a family member. The staff member does not see any conflicts about seeing you in a professional capacity. In fact, they may have actually been referred by one of the physicians in your practice who also is the staff member's personal physician. Most psychologists will be very uncomfortable being placed in this role. While there are different perspectives on the optimal response to this situation, the author has evolved a policy in which he indicates that he will meet with the person once to assist in referring them to appropriate services. Providing a brief explanation to the referring physician and staff member about the reasons for not seeing them as a patient is typically respected. Discussing psychologists' ethical guidelines around this issue will assure the staff member that you are not rejecting them or questioning the referring physician's professional judgment.

Because of their specialized expertise, the psychologist may periodically receive requests to address personnel issues. For example, one of the physicians in your group pulls you into an exam room, shuts the door, and says:

> Julie, the nurse in our practice is become as been coming in later and later. She's making more mistakes – she's misreading blood pressures and writing the patient's weight incorrectly. Yesterday, I think I smelled alcohol on her breath. I'm worried about patient care but I know that Julie's having some marital problems. What should I do? Can *you* talk to her?

The focus of the request may also be a conflict between physicians in the practice. Four of Dr. Jones' colleagues descend on your office to vent about Dr. Smith, a practice colleague with whom they have been having ongoing problems.

These are obviously difficult issues – particularly when patient welfare may be compromised. Modeling a somewhat detached, nonreactive stance, as suggested by Caplan, is, by itself, often helpful. In addition there are several other guidelines useful for these situations: First, rather than agreeing with the complainant(s), it is helpful to ask how the colleague or staff member's behavior is impacting them personally. Second, do not take sides in the conflict but ask questions to help clarify the situation. Third, if providing an opinion or making a recommendation about how to address the problem person, phrase it in general terms rather than specific to the individual in question. (While I don't know enough about the situation to say anything specific about Dr. Jones, often, when people are going through a divorce, their behavior can be erratic for a few months.) At the same time, the psychologist should be supportive of the distressed consulting physician who has sought them out. If nothing else, the discussion may provide those concerned with a different perspective on the situation. Often, since physicians are fairly good problem solvers, some resolution may occur simply from talking privately with the psychologist who summarizes and reflects the key issues.

Conversations About Patients and Office Gossip

Psychologists, because of their sensitivity to interpersonal boundaries, can provide useful role modeling to their medical colleagues and office staff in discussing patients. As suggested above, the psychologist is, at some level, providing consultation for the entire practice – not simply the patients. It is important to consider this role when interacting with physicians and medical staff. A desire to "fit in" as a member of the health care team should not override the psychologist's professionalism. Because of the clinic's intense pace, high volume of patients, as well as the physician's anxiety about missing a life-threatening diagnosis coupled with their strong sense of responsibility, and because medicine is a culture with its own "ingroup" norms, there is a tendency to talk about patients in a way that blames them for their illness. This blaming is also likely to be influenced by the interaction between physicians who feel a responsibility to cure patients with chronic illness that has been brought about by an unhealthy lifestyle as well as the frustration in searching for a diagnosis in patients with nonspecific symptoms. This ingroup – outgroup dynamic helps reduce anxiety by increasing group cohesion (Waskett, 1995). Blaming the victim for their illness and even their death absolves the health care professional of responsibility and reduces their anxiety about illness and death because they would never engage in similar behavior.

Psychologists, because they may know particularly personal patient information, can have "special" status by sharing "original nugget(s) of gossip" (Waskett, 1999, p. 123). Particularly when they are relatively new to the primary care setting and often experiencing anxiety and doubt about professional competence in this challenging role, psychologists may be at risk for sharing information unprofessionally. This action is obviously an ethical breach but also communicates to physician colleagues and other health care staff that seemingly confidential information – including possible information that these other professionals may have disclosed to the psychologist – is not managed respectfully. To maintain this integrity, the psychologist should avoid jokes and/or gossip about patients. In addition, it also means that when discussing patients with physicians and office staff, the psychologist maintains a respectful, business like tone. The psychologist who feels that they are being pulled into gossip or participating in a discussion in which patients are referred to in derogatory terms should ask themselves how they would feel if the person being discussed overheard the exchange.

Physicians sometimes use dismissive terms to deal with patients whom they find very frustrating. This may be particularly true for physicians still in training as residents or medical students. With minimal professional experience, there is the added burden of being evaluated by faculty physicians and peers. There may be a tendency to manage this distress by using derogatory terms for patients and seeing them as different from of the rest of us (Waskett, 1999). Hearing terms such as GOMER (an acronym for Get Out of My Emergency Room), "train wreck" (for patients with multiple significant medical problems), or 'psycho" (describing patients who are irrational) is typically a sign that the physician is frustrated, experiencing helplessness and/or hopelessness, or is simply overworked. By making the patient the target, it provides a useful, albeit unconscious repository for these feelings. Stein (1986) suggests that these terms also reveal physicians' explanatory models for patients – a concept discussed further in Chapter 10. These physician-held models are not biomedical and move these challenging patients from the cognitive category of "sick" to a category of patients who may not have bona fide medical illness or whose illness resulted from the patient's voluntarily chosen unhealthy lifestyle (Stein, 1986). Psychologists, hearing these terms while gathering information about a referral, should take these utterances as a likely sign of a difficult physician-patient relationship.

Clinical Management of Referrals

When seeing a patient for the first time, the psychologist should remember to clarify their role. The psychologist should stress that they are in a consultant relationship with the primary care physician who referred the patient. As a general rule, it is helpful for psychologists to begin the patient encounters by explaining the referral information they have received from the physician. (It's my understanding that Dr. Johnson asked you to see me today because of headaches. It sounded as if Dr. Johnson was concerned that perhaps stress was playing a role in your headaches. Is that your understanding?) In other instances, the psychologist may not have information about the patient – time pressures may have prevented the physician from talking directly with psychologist or an updated chart may not be available. In these instances, it is useful to begin by conveying the understanding that the patient was referred by their physician but requesting clarification as to the reasons. (I was unable to talk with Dr. Smith before our meeting, today. I do understand that she suggested that you see me. What is your understanding of the reasons that you are seeing me today?) Psychologists should also inform the patient that information will be shared with their primary care physician. If the psychologist is not part of the same practice as the physician, an appropriate release of information should be obtained.

In dealing with somatoform patients, the psychologist should be particularly careful about how they begin the interview. Even when a thorough medical workup has been conducted and organic disease has been ruled out, the psychologist should not expect that the patient necessarily agrees that the problem is psychological in nature. In order to develop rapport with these patients, it is helpful to ask them to describe and explain the history of their illness including previous treatment. It is also critical to ask the patient how they feel about about being referred to a psychologist. As mentioned in the previous chapter, do not assume that the patient views their physical symptoms as psychologically based. After obtaining a thorough account of the history and the patient's perspective on their symptoms, the psychologist should verbally summarize their understanding of the patient's concerns. Only after there is a mutual understanding of these issues, should questions about the role of psychosocial factors be introduced. However, as described in Chapter 2, rather than focusing on how environmental and psychosocial stress may impact the patient's physical complaints, it is more helpful to ask how the physical complaints impact their psychological, social, and physical well-being. By not challenging the reality of the physical complaints, patients' defensiveness will be reduced and a fuller picture of the relationship between their symptoms and various aspects of the patient's life can be obtained.

The psychologist, as a general rule, should not rely exclusively on the patient history obtained by another provider. At the outset, the psychologist should indicate to the patient that they may be asking somewhat similar questions as the physician but always find it helpful to obtain information directly from the patient. Patients typically respond very positively to this explanation and will rarely be irritated about having to repeat aspects of their history.

Medical Conditions

Psychologists are not physicians. However, psychologists should have basic knowledge about common conditions and reasons that patients are seen in primary care. These range from childhood immunizations to acute upper respiratory infections. In particular, psychologists should have knowledge about chronic illness such as asthma, chronic obstructive pulmonary disease, and hypertension. Knowledge about common therapies for these conditions as well as medical tests and basic laboratory values associated with them (e.g., hemoglobin A-1 C as a marker for diabetic control over approximately the past 3 months) will also enhance patient care and help address adherence.

Primary care physicians are typically happy to explain aspects of clinical medicine to psychologists who demonstrate interest. It is the author's experience that physicians often assume that the psychologist knows more about medicine than they did actually do. Other ways to pick up relevant information are to attend conferences and to read clinical primary care textbooks such as those used by medical students (e.g., Mengel & Schwiebert, 2009).

Communication

Communication about patient care takes multiple forms. There is formal written medical chart documentation, informal "curbside" consultation in which the physician approaches the psychologist to discuss the patient, and formal consultation with a typed consultation note and/or letter. As noted earlier, written communication should be brief. A typical consultation note is about 1 1/2 pages and should be organized with frequent subheadings to model the format that is used by other specialist consultants (Searight et al., 2004). Finally, the written note should include a very concise summary of the patient's condition, a formal diagnosis, and a plan for treatment. It is important to remember that the psychologist is not the primary professional responsible for the patient – that role is held by the referring physician.

Some mental health practitioners have developed referral sheets for physicians to complete when sending a patient to them. This approach is helpful because the process of completing a formal referral often helps the physician clarify the clinical question that they would like to have addressed. In addition, by having a place on the form for the psychologist to give their impressions of the patient immediately after the consultation visit, referral feedback can be expedited. However, even with the referral sheet, unfocused questions are likely to persist. There will still be physicians whose referral question is merely "evaluate patient."

For patient privacy and welfare, it is important that the psychologist consider the types of information to be formally documented. When writing or dictating information in a medical chart, the psychologist should always assume that the chart will be read by many other people including the referring physician, nurses, X-ray technicians, insurance reviewers, hospital administrators, attorneys, government agencies, and often patients, themselves. Mental health information often requires a specific patient release form and is not covered by a general release of the medical record. However, at the same time, a records clerk may not be aware of this distinction and mistakenly, but routinely, send the psychologist's notes along with medical notes to third parties. A useful strategy used by some clinics is to establish a separate section of the medical record specific for mental health information. A related approach has been to use a different color of paper for mental health notes.

Because of the probability of third-party disclosure and particularly in inpatient settings where a large number of allied health professionals have access to the record, psychologists should carefully consider the content of their notes. If during a psychological assessment of an adult female hospitalized for diabetic complications, a sexual abuse history is disclosed, the psychologist should carefully consider whether this information is necessary for other professionals working with the patient. While it may be helpful to a primary care physician, obstetrician, or gynecologist to know about this history, it is probably not essential that hospital administrators, insurance companies, or laboratory technicians know these details. In these situations, the author will usually indicate in the written chart note that a specific stressful event has occurred in the patient's life, but to protect privacy, the actual nature of the event is not disclosed in writing. Professionals who may need to know this information to better carry out patient care can be informed verbally. Finally, if the patient does seek to have their mental health information disclosed to third parties, the psychologist should inform the patient if the psychologist's notes include anything particularly sensitive, embarrassing, prejudicial, or otherwise unhelpful to the patient. The patient may withdraw consent to send the information, or the psychologist may send a summary with sensitive, unnecessary, data removed.

Conclusion

Practicing in a primary care environment requires a number of skills in which few psychologists are formally trained. Most currently practicing primary care psychologists received "on-the-job training." The majority of the patients seen by the psychologist will be on referral from primary care physicians. In some practices, psychologists require that the patients be referred by their physician and do not accept self-referred patients who have not seen their physician in the past 4–6 months. This provides some assurance that any medical problems have been diagnosed and are being addressed. The psychologist is not the patient's primary health care provider. Psychologists, however, because of their training, do bring a unique perspective to interpersonal issues in primary care practices as well as physician-patient issues that may prompt referrals.

Chapter 4

When You Hear Hoofbeats, Think of Horses – Not Zebras

Applied Epidemiology, Brief Assessment, and Population-Oriented Intervention

Overview

As the previous chapter emphasized, efficiency is paramount in primary care. When evaluating patients, physicians often operate according to a number of implicit decisional rules or algorithms. These are generally based upon both their experience in a particular setting as well as knowledge of probabilities that symptoms indicate a particular condition. At the same time, periodic, but infrequent, misdiagnosis in which a relatively benign condition is incorrectly diagnosed, while a more serious one is actually present, reminds physicians to be aware that there are exceptions to these implicit cognitive rules.

After a brief review of epidemiology, several examples of using population-based data with psychiatric disorders will be described. With this familiar territory as a background, the focus will then turn to the comorbidity of many medical conditions, health risk factors, and mental health problems. A number of examples will be provided to highlight how knowledge of prevalence, incidence, and comorbidity patterns in the general population as well as in the primary care sector, more specifically, can help psychologists evaluate patients with greater efficiency. The next section focuses upon psychological screening tools that can be applied to primary care. A sampling of useful instruments is presented. However, this section is immediately followed by a caveat about the dangers of relying upon population-based or screening measures, alone for diagnosis.

Because of the sheer quantity of patients in primary care and the high prevalence of psychiatric problems as well as associated behavioral risk issues, interventions may have somewhat different goals than complete behavior change. Rather than "curing," valued outcomes in primary care are symptom reduction, improved daily functioning as well as improving health, and reducing, rather than eliminating, risk behavior. Population benefits of this approach are described with evidence-based examples.

Finally, several interventions, such as computerized therapies, are presented as examples of brief, population-oriented interventions that do have limited empirical support. While evidence will be presented in the chapters which follow on specific intervention techniques, the conclusion of the current chapter will examine this issue somewhat more broadly and hopefully leave the reader reassured that brief treatment can have significant impact.

Review of Epidemiology

Epidemiology is the study of the causes and distribution of health conditions and risk factors across time and space in various social groups (Coreil, 2010). Epidemiology's overall objective is to determine factors that are associated with the incidence and prevalence of disease. Incidence, the number of new cases of the condition per unit of time, is helpful when the goal is to understand changes in rates of new diseases. Prevalence, more commonly used in psychiatry, addresses the total number of cases in a population at any particular point in time.

Determining a causal relationship between a risk factor and an outcome is best achieved through a longitudinal study. Because of the time and expense required, cross-sectional and case control studies are much more common. As a result, much of epidemiology centers on established associations between risk factors or between risk factors and clinical conditions, rather than clearly established causal pathways. For the primary care clinician, who is attempting to use all available information for efficient assessment and treatment recommendations, knowledge of an association between factors, rather than a clearly delineated causal model, is typically sufficient. For example, there is a strong relationship between cigarette smoking and major depressive symptoms. While it is likely that nicotine is particularly reinforcing to individuals with preexisting dysphoric mood and fatigue because of its stimulant properties, depressive symptoms may actually emerge after the smoking habit is well entrenched. In either case, knowledge of the association will remind psychologists treating patients for smoking cessation to assess for depression and also, conversely, to remember that patients with depression are more likely to have health risk behavior such as smoking.

In examining the psychological and behavioral factors associated with health risks such as unprotected sex, cigarette smoking, auto accidents, and obesity, one of the most useful sources is the Behavioral Risk Factor Surveillance System (BRFS). For example, in 2008, 35% of Michigan residents were considered overweight with an additional 31% considered obese (Centers for Disease Control, 2009). A version of the BRFS targeted to high school students, provides data about sexual behavior and risks for sexually transmitted diseases. This information is particularly useful for psychologists who see or consult on adolescent patients – it provides a benchmark against which to compare behaviors commonly assessed in well-teenager exams that are of concern to physicians and parents. Nationwide, 7% of high school students report having sexual intercourse before age 13, with 15% of high school students having had four or more sexual partners, and 23%

having used alcohol or drugs before their last sexual encounter (Centers for Disease Control, 2009).

Why a Population Orientation Is Important for Primary Care

Primary care practices are responsible for a small community of patients. The average primary care physician may have multiple thousand patients in their practice pool. With considerable evidence of high rates of psychiatric disorder as well as lifestyle factors such as obesity and smoking responsible for much chronic illness in the primary care population, traditional individually focused, extended treatment is impractical. A focus on individuals, accompanied by a view that treatment should continue until the individual is completely symptom-free, is impractical given the level of risk behaviors and psychiatric symptoms in an average medical practice. The prevalence of the condition, the number of people in the population who are ill, reflects the upper bound of symptoms or risk factors in a specific population. This relationship has been found for hypertension, heart disease, gambling addiction, and other mental health conditions. Because these conditions are very common, symptoms and risk factors are actually distributed across the entire population rather than clustered in high-risk subgroups (Huppert, 2009).

One of the best studied examples, alcohol use, has been the focus of a number of brief interventions in primary care (Babor et al., 1999). It has been found that average alcohol consumption in a particular region is strongly associated with problem drinking prevalence in that area. Because the problem behavior or symptom, in this case, drinking, is highly prevalent, a small reduction in the average overall consumption – particularly in light or moderate drinkers – can result in a significant decrease in prevalence rates of problem drinking (defined by a consumption level greater than a set criterion number of drinks per week – typically ranging from 14 to 21 depending on the standard employed). Therefore, if a large number of people in the subpopulation consume one or two fewer alcoholic drinks per week, problem drinking in the population as a whole will be reduced by a greater magnitude than if intervention efforts simply targeted individual problem drinkers (Huppert, 2009). When examining broad-based psychological distress, Huppert (2009) found that for every one point drop in the symptom score on the General Health Questionnaire (GHQ), there was a 7% drop in the prevalence of mental health disorders.

The High Prevalence of Psychiatric Conditions in the General Population

Physicians routinely use probability-based heuristics when evaluating patients. One of the most basic and useful dimensions is the prevalence of a condition in the general population. Physicians implicitly consider high base rate (horses) rather than low prevalence (zebras) conditions when evaluating patients with new symptoms (hoof beats).

Internationally, mental illness is currently the second leading cause of disability in the world. According to the World Health Organization (WHO, 2003) mental health problems have become one of the primary causes of lost workforce productivity worldwide. At best, only half of those with psychiatric problems receive any type of professional assistance (WHO, 2003). At any given time, one of four Americans meets criteria for a mental health condition.

Prevalence rates – particularly of mood and anxiety disorders – are increasing in industrialized countries and will be reflected in the primary care population. In examining 12-month prevalence rates, Kessler, Chiu, Demler, and Walters (2005) found that up to 30% of the general US population met Diagnostic and Statistical Manual of Mental Disorders (DSM) criteria for at least one mental disorder within the past year (Kessler et al., 2005). Nearly 10% met diagnostic criteria for a mood disorder with 18% exhibiting symptoms of an anxiety disorder. Of note, approximately 6% met criteria for two psychiatric disorders with another 6% meeting criteria for three or more conditions during the 12-month time frame (Kessler et al., 2005).

Demographic features associated with differing prevalences of psychiatric conditions in the general population are also useful when conducting time-limited assessments. Factors protecting against psychiatric illness include male gender, non-Hispanic black or Hispanic ethnicity, being married, having a college education, higher income, and rural place of residence (Kessler et al., 2005). When categorizing psychiatric illnesses into internalizing conditions (e.g., major depressive disorder) or externalizing conditions (e.g., antisocial personality disorder or attention deficit hyperactivity disorder (AD/HD)), demographic risk factors were found be associated with each type of condition. Internalizing disorders were more common among married women with higher levels of education who were suburban residents. Externalizing disorders were more common among younger males of Hispanic background living in rural areas. Those with comorbid internalizing disorders, such as coexisting depression and anxiety, were more likely to be female, previously married, and suburban residents. Those who had both internalizing and externalizing conditions, simultaneously, were more likely to be younger, married, males residing in a nonrural area (Kessler et al., 2005).

Knowledge of Risk Factors Improves Clinical Reasoning

Family Pedigree

Family history is a standard part of a primary care physician's evaluation of a new patient. For example, interviews with family physicians, general internists, and gynecologists found that these physicians routinely obtained a family history regarding cancer risk. This was most commonly done with new patients with nearly all physicians indicating that this history was standard (Wood, Stockdale, & Flynn, 2008). Ideally the history includes the type of cancer affecting family members and age of disease onset for first- and second-degree relatives on both the maternal and paternal sides of the family. It is estimated that about 20% of primary care patients will have a positive family history for cancer. Similar family pedigrees are gathered for cardiovascular diseases such as myocardial infarction

(MI; heart attack) and stroke. Clinically, physicians use family pedigree information for informal risk stratification of patients as well as to reassure some patients and encourage early screening for others.

Genetic Risk Factors for Psychiatric Conditions

Mental health professionals are aware of the heritability of many forms of psychiatric illness but may not always apply these probabilities in clinical assessment. Psychiatric conditions with well-established genetic risk factors include panic disorder, drug abuse, schizophrenia, bipolar disorder, and autism. For example, among identical twins, concordance rates for panic disorder were 24% and 11% in dizygotic twins (Kendler, Neale, Kessler, Heath, & Eaves; 1993). Schizophrenia has been particularly well studied for genetic factors. Children whose biological parents have been diagnosed with schizophrenia are 10–15 times more likely to develop the condition themselves (Susser & Schwartz, 2006). Concordance rates for identical twins are 48% with children of two schizophrenic parents having a 46% likelihood of developing the disorder. Schizophrenia concordance rates for fraternal twins are 17% with a 13% likelihood of children developing the condition if one parent has schizophrenia (Comer, 2010).

While genetic data are more difficult to interpret, alcohol abuse also appears to have a hereditary component. Studies of identical twins have found a concordance rate of 54% with a corresponding concordance rate of 28% for alcohol abuse in fraternal twins (Comer, 2010). However, while it is clear that genetics do play a role in the development of alcohol and other substance abuse problems, it has been difficult to determine the relative influence of genetics versus environment in these conditions.

Nongenetic Risk Factors for Mental Health Conditions: Actuarial Reasoning

Mental health professionals are generally aware of multiple causal models for specific psychiatric conditions. However, from an actuarial perspective, there are a number of factors that increase the likelihood of developing a psychiatric diagnosis in which specific factors raise the risk of developing the condition (e.g., borderline personality disorder and parenting style) in the absence of well-established causal mechanisms. From an assessment perspective, a clear causal pathway is less important than the fact that a particular social, environmental, or personal characteristic increases the likelihood of a particular disorder being present. An analogy is the "good student" discounts given by auto insurance companies to high school-aged drivers. While the exact mechanism relating a "B" average grade point to a reduced rate of auto accidents has not been well articulated, the relationship between these two factors has been consistently demonstrated at a population level. The relationship is of sufficient magnitude and consistency that these data form the basis for computing auto insurance premiums for younger drivers. This approach is the essence of actuarial reasoning – an approach that can be adapted to primary care to assist in efficient clinical assessment.

Risk factors continue to be discovered for the development of Alzheimer's disease. These include a history of a head injury, lower level of formal education, aluminum exposure, female sex, psychiatric history, as well as the presumed genetic contribution of having a first-degree relative with dementia (Zimmerman, Ahsan, & Susser, 2006).

Social epidemiology has found moderate to large associations between various social factors such as poverty, rapid changes in the economic status of a community, and residential segregation by race and the probability of health events such as heart attacks (Berkman, 2004). While not as well established in the United States, there is some evidence in European studies that rates of severe psychiatric distress – such as schizophrenia – may be significantly higher among immigrant groups. Of note, rates appear to be even higher in second-generation family members of immigrants from areas such as Morocco or the Caribbean (Susser & Schwartz, 2006). In the United States, frequent job changes are a marker of elevated risk for psychiatric symptoms (Cherry, 1976).

Natural experiments can also provide useful information about risk factors associated with psychiatric symptoms (Susser & Schwartz, 2006). For example, among children living in poverty in the rural south, there was a major decrease in psychiatric symptomatology when a tribal casino opened in the area and the level of poverty was reduced. A natural experiment involving threatening events – terrorist attacks or severe natural disasters – has established risk factors for developing posttraumatic stress disorder (PTSD). It is important to recognize that the majority of those exposed to traumatic events do not develop PTSD and that their symptoms typically fall to subclinical levels within approximately 30 days after exposure to a traumatic event. However, those who are more likely to continue to manifest clinically significant symptoms are those with previous trauma experiences, psychiatric histories such as depressive disorder, female gender, and those with ongoing litigation.

It is also important to consider cohort effects (Morris, 1975) when applying epidemiological findings to clinical assessment. One example of a significant cohort effect is the diagnosis of Attention Deficit/Hyperactivity Disorder (AD/HD) in adulthood. Early studies of adult outcomes of childhood ADHD estimated that approximately 30% of children with the disorder continued to have pronounced ADHD symptoms in adulthood (Weiss & Hechtman, 1993). More recent investigations suggest that up to 70% of adults with childhood histories of the condition manifest adult symptoms. One likely reason for this pattern is the change in diagnostic criteria for ADHD from the DSM-III to the DSM-IV. The earlier diagnostic criteria for ADD, as it was called in the DSM-III, emphasized hyperactivity with less emphasis on inattentive symptoms. The more recent DSM-IV diagnostic formulation gave equal weight to inattention and impulsivity/hyperactivity such that milder forms of the syndrome now qualified for the diagnosis (Searight & McLaren, 1998).

Health Risk Behaviors: "Where There's Smoke, There's Fire"

Health risk behaviors tend to cluster – persons engaging in one harmful habit often have several other risks. Heavy drinkers – men who consume 12 or more alcoholic drinks per week and/or five or more drinks on one occasion, and women consuming nine or more drinks per week and/or four or more on one occasion – are more likely to smoke and significantly less likely to engage in regular exercise (Rosal, Ockene, Hurley, & Reiff, 2000). Demographic characteristics associated with a larger number of health risk behaviors include male gender, a lower level of formal education, unmarried status, and unemployment or employment in a blue collar job. When patients engaging in multiple unhealthy behaviors were asked directly, smoking and sedentary status were more likely to be perceived as problematic compared with excess alcohol use which was often minimized. Rosal et al. (2000) suggest that by beginning with the patient's priority behavior – increased physical activity and decreasing or eliminating cigarettes – early success may make these patients more amenable to subsequently reducing their alcohol use.

Major depressive disorder is also common among cigarette smokers. Some studies have placed the prevalence rates of depression among smokers at 20–30%. Of the three factors associated with initiation of smoking in adolescence – the age at which most people begin the habit – two are interpersonal and one is psychiatric. Having parents who smoke as well as a number of peers who smoke are well-known risk factors. Many clinicians are unaware that depression is the third risk factor for smoking initiation (Searight, 1992). The presence of major depressive disorder also plays a role in smoking cessation. Patients who are depressed are far less likely to be successful in their attempts to quit smoking. It has been hypothesized that the typical dysphoria and irritability associated with nicotine withdrawal is particularly pronounced among smokers with preexisting depressive symptoms. Treating the depression before initiating smoking cessation is a strategy that should be seriously considered.

Psychiatric Symptoms in Primary Care

Psychologists should expect to find higher rates of most psychiatric disorders among primary care patients. Depression is present in approximately 21% of primary care patients based on 12-month prevalence data with 22% of female and approximately 17% of male patients exhibiting depressive symptoms in the past year (Cwikel, Zilber, Feinson, & Lerner, 2008). Of note, anxiety disorders were about equally common in primary care as in the general population. This pattern can be explained by the fact that the most common anxiety disorder, specific phobia, is rarely a focus of treatment in primary care and is often self-managed by patients through maintaining environments that do not include the phobic stimulus.

Of note, subthreshold conditions such as nonspecific cognitive impairment, depressive symptoms that did not reach the threshold of DSM criteria, and panic attacks affected approximately 15% of both male and female primary care patients. Some authors have suggested that psychiatric symptoms, such as depression and anxiety, be viewed similarly to blood pressure (Brugha, 2002). In examining the distribution of the symptoms of depression in the general population, the resulting pattern is continuous with no indication of a clearly defined clinical and nonclinical group (Brugha, 2002). Population-based investigators have also questioned whether the requirement of five symptoms of 2 weeks duration found in the DSM-IV is meaningfully tied to health outcomes. A population-based study using the General Health Questionnaire found that 7-year survival was best predicted by the entire distribution of scores in a given population rather than an arbitrary high or low subgroup (Huppert & Whittington, 2003).

A similar issue has been raised with respect to the relationship between memory functioning and dementia. In examining performance on a prospective memory task (sealing and initialing an envelope with a 10-minute delay between instructions and task initiation), it was found that 54% of the population between 65 and 90 performed the task correctly. Of note, 68% of those between 65 and 69 performed correctly but only 19% of those aged 90 and above were successful. The authors conclude that short-term recall, as assessed by their prospective memory task, is deficient in a high percentage of the elderly population. The prospective memory task was particularly sensitive to mild early dementia with only 8% of that early dementia performing the task correctly. The authors express concern that the majority of those in the mild early dementia group (85%) were living at home with 20% living alone (Huppert, Johnson, & Nickson, 2000).

The existence of broad-based memory impairment is of concern for patient safety. Again, the primary care psychologist should consider the impact of mild cognitive impairment on daily living abilities when evaluating older patients.

These subclinical conditions are noteworthy in that they seem to be associated with increased physical disability and impaired functioning (Oxman & Sengupta, 2002). As noted in Chapter 2, psychiatric symptoms, rather than formal syndromes, are best understood as existing on a curvilinear continuum with a direct relationship between number of symptoms and health outcomes. When examined from a risk factor perspective, depressive and anxiety symptoms demonstrate strong associations with behaviors such as smoking, increased body mass index (BMI), alcohol use, and sedentary lifestyle. While some of the variance in health outcomes such as cardiovascular death, hypertension, and diabetes are associated with these risk behaviors, psychiatric symptoms have consistently demonstrated an independent association with morbidity and mortality (Denollet et al., 2009).

It is important to recognize that these are associations rather than causal factors. For example, increased medical burden, poorer subjective health, and lower levels of social support have been found to be associated with longer-term outcomes for major depressive disorder (Lyness et al., 2006). However it is difficult to determine if health and social support lead to mood disorders or whether the presence of mood disorder symptoms adversely impacts these other two variables. From the perspective of primary care assessment, causal relationships are less important than the associations themselves – again, these are "red flags" for the clinician. When one of these factors is present, there is increased likelihood that other risk behaviors or psychiatric symptoms are present. On the other hand, protective factors for mental health conditions in the primary care setting include older age (65–75 years), higher levels of education, being married, having an adequate income, and full-time employment (Cwikel et al., 2008).

Approximately 20% of US adults have a recent history of alcohol abuse (Fleming, Manwell, Barry, & Johnson, 1998). In terms of the health impact, alcohol use has been the subject of multiple primary care population-based and early intervention studies.

One of the difficulties with alcohol use is that patients tend to underreport their consumption. Research has suggested that patients are reasonably accurate in reporting the number of specific drinking episodes within a time frame (number of days that they consumed alcohol in the past month) but the amount consumed on each occasion does tend to be underreported. There are also suggestions that patients consuming alcohol in greater quantities are more likely to consult their primary care physician (Searight, 1992). Because of the tendency to underreport use, efforts have been made to examine the types of symptoms that patients with alcohol are likely to present in primary care. A linear relationship has been established between nonspecific physical symptoms – tremulousness, insomnia, and upset stomach – and alcohol abuse. Gastrointestinal symptoms, in particular, appear to be particularly sensitive. When three nonspecific GI symptoms were present, there was at least a 25% likelihood that the patient was abusing alcohol (Malla & Merskey, 1987; Searight, 1992).

Of interest, health risks of alcohol use also appear to be continuous rather than categorical. Individuals consuming more than 20 g of alcohol per day (a standard alcoholic drink is 12–14 g of alcohol) had a risk of liver cirrhosis that was 2.2 times greater than that of the general population. For every 10 g of alcohol consumed on a daily basis, systolic and diastolic blood pressures increased by 1–2 mm Hg (Fleming et al., 1998).

Comorbidity of Medical and Psychiatric Conditions

Most psychologists are aware of psychiatric conditions that have high comorbidities. For example, among children, AD/HD often coexists with conduct disorder and oppositional defiant disorder. In adults, there is often a strong relationship between anxiety disorders and major depressive disorder. For example, among adults with obsessive compulsive disorder, rates of major depressive disorder may be as high as 40% (Tukel, Polat, Ozdemir, Aksut, & Turksoy, 2002). This knowledge of co-occurring conditions is helpful in the assessment process since a diagnosis of one disorder substantially increases the likelihood that the patient will have a common coexisting condition at a prevalence rate far above the general population.

In the primary care setting, similar patterns occur with the coexistence of medical and mental health conditions. Chronic illness is a major risk factor for depressive illness. Among physicians, the presence of conditions such as hypertension, type II diabetes, and rheumatoid arthritis may make it more difficult for them to accurately detect, formally diagnose, and treat depression (Ani et al., 2009). However, it is clear that chronic illness is associated with substantially higher rates of major depressive disorder with 25–50% of chronically ill patients having it as a comorbid condition.

Comorbid major depressive disorder is increasingly recognized as a predictor of later morbidity and mortality. The relationship between psychological distress and health outcomes, including cardiovascular death, hypertension, and type II diabetes, has indicated that psychiatric symptoms predict death and disability apart from shared variance with risk factors. Major depressive disorder is an independent predictor of subsequent heart failure after the patient has sustained an initial episode (May et al., 2009). Again, the practical significance is that post-MI patients should be routinely screened for the presence of major depressive disorder and secondarily for anxiety disorders. Patients with chronic lower back pain also have significantly elevated rates of major depressive illness. Research to date suggests that depression may play a role in the pathway from acute lower back pain to chronic pain. In these patients, depression appears to occur after the onset of the pain and is likely to amplify and increase disability (Searight, 1999). Tension headaches, a very common presenting complaint in primary care, are also markers for psychiatric distress with up to 50% of these patients having major depressive and/or anxiety disorder (Bair, Robinson, Katon, & Kroenke, 2002; The Italian Collaborative Group, 2002).

Substance abuse – either in the form of narcotic abuse/dependence or alcohol abuse – is also commonly associated with chronic lower back pain. Again, detecting a substance abuse condition in these patients is important because the rebound from prescription medication may serve to intensify the pain. Additionally, alcohol is well known as a depressant and may further contribute to inactivity among these patients which, in turn, increases reported pain.

Among older adults, at least a third have chronic joint pain. With increased age, arthritis increases from 2 to 10 times between the ages of 30 and 60 (He et al., 2008). In the United States, an estimated 9–10% of those with rheumatoid arthritis have comorbid major depressive disorder. When compared with comparably aged persons without arthritis, those with the condition are twice as likely to meet criteria for dysthymic disorder (He et al., 2008). Additionally, when compared with patients without arthritis, those with arthritis were twice as likely to have an anxiety disorder.

As noted above, short-term memory deficits are highly prevalent in the over age 65 population. Currently, research is being conducted on early predictors of Alzheimer's disease. Early detection is important for several reasons including planning for later care giving and initiating medications which may temporarily prevent cognitive decline. These medications tend to be most helpful to patients in early stages of Alzheimer's and may initially reduce cognitive decline by the equivalent of about 6 months. At present, short-term memory loss, along with difficulties in numerical computation and problem solving, appear to be particularly sensitive early indicators of the condition. Of note, the presence of major depressive disorder in early stages of Alzheimer's disease is also common and is associated with poorer cognitive functioning.

Primary care psychologists are likely to be able to conduct more efficient assessment when cognizant of the relationship between medical and psychiatric illness. As will be discussed further, aggressively treating mental health problems among the chronically ill will improve medical outcomes and reduce further morbidity.

The Impact of Mental Health Conditions on Medical Problems

In addition to raising a diagnostic flag for psychologists, the presence of a psychiatric condition directly affects the course and severity of the medical condition and vice versa (Katon, 2003). For example, diabetic patients with untreated major depressive disorder have a higher rate of diabetic complications such as retinopathy which may result in eventual blindness. Major depressive disorder is also a very potent predictor of morbidity and mortality for cardiovascular disease. For example, patients who have experienced a MI may be twice as likely to have a second infarction if untreated major depressive disorders present (Van Melle et al., 2004). Rehospitalization for congestive heart failure is also strongly predicted by the presence of major depressive disorder. Among elderly patients who are undergoing surgery for hip fracture, the presence or absence of major depressive disorder is a more potent predictor of whether the patient will be walking at 1 year (Mossey, Mutran, Knott, & Craik, 1989). As noted above, arthritis is often associated with elevated levels of anxiety and mood disorder. Among persons with arthritis, treating depression leads to better levels of physical functioning and activity level (Lin et al., 2003).

Implications of Psychiatric-Medical Comorbidities for the Primary Care Psychologist

There are significant clinical implications of this pattern for psychologists. First, research suggests that physicians seem to be less likely to diagnose psychiatric disorders in patients with multiple physical complaints. This may be a function of the need to prioritize complaints from most to least serious in response to time constraints. Primary care physicians typically require multiple patient visits to disentangle the relative role of depression or anxiety versus organic illness in causing relatively nonspecific symptoms such as fatigue, insomnia, poor appetite, dizziness, diffuse muscle tension, and pain, as well reports or abnormal bodily sensations such as heart rate and respiration. Psychiatric conditions are often given serious consideration only after serious, potentially life-threatening medical illness is ruled out. It is certainly understandable that a physician would want to be sure that the patient's chest pain is not angina reflective of heart disease before diagnosing panic disorder. While the exact relationship between medical illness and psychiatric diagnoses has not always been well explicated, one very practical conclusion from research is that the presence of major depressive disorder makes it three times as likely that the patient will be nonadherent with a chronic illness regimen (DiMatteo, 2004). If the psychologist is able to diagnose and recommend treatment for these patients, the patient's overall health status is likely to be better which is also likely to improve their relationship with their physician.

Screening: Efficient Diagnostic Interviewing

In conducting primary care diagnostic interviews, psychologists' efficiency can be improved by using informal algorithms such that the absence of symptoms typically associated with a given condition temporarily rules out particular diagnoses and the presence of a particular symptom leads to more detailed questioning. For example, patients who report no changes in sleeping habits, deny dysphoric or angry-irritable mood and can describe several areas of life satisfaction in an animated tone are less likely to be depressed. Similarly, in asking patients about fear and anxiety, those who describe enduring anxiety states that do not vary throughout the day are much more likely to have generalized anxiety rather than panic disorder. When evaluating a child for possible AD/HD, a child who is performing well academically, and is not exhibiting any behavior problems in the classroom but is demonstrating some disruptive behavior at home, is far less likely to have that condition. Again, there are unusual variations on presentations of most clinical conditions, and if continued symptom focused interviewing and history-taking does not lead to a consistent diagnosis, the interviewer may need to ask further about some of these earlier symptoms or vary the style of questioning.

Demographic information should also be used to cognitively "triage" patients into higher and lower probability diagnostic categories. For example, a 70-year-old male presenting with acute psychotic symptoms who has no prior mental health history and has been functioning well until recently is unlikely to have a functional psychiatric condition such as schizophrenia. The possibility of a physiologically based condition such as delirium is much more likely. Similarly, a 45-year-old male who has been referred to you for "depression" that has had a history of multiple incarcerations may be depressed but the probability of antisocial personality disorder should also be high on the list of diagnostic possibilities. Finally, there is other social information that often can be used to reduce the range of probable diagnoses. A patient referred by their physician for "adjustment problems," who is receiving Supplemental Social Security Income (disability payments) for a psychiatric condition is likely to have a much more severe condition than the referral suggests. Primary care psychologists, similar to primary care physicians, should always be aware that while reasoning based on probabilities will be accurate a good deal of the time, there are exceptions. These exceptions can have life-threatening consequences. This issue will be explored further in a later section of this chapter.

Useful Psychiatric Screening Instruments for Primary Care

Most psychologists are familiar with a range of self-report screening instruments. In the past 10–15 years, a number of these tools have been developed specifically for primary care. Others, such as the Beck Depression Inventory (BDI) and the Mini-Mental Status Examination (MMSE), while not specifically developed for this context, are time efficient and have population norms. The scales listed below have reasonably well-established reliability and validity and are of two general types – broad-based screening tools and narrower diagnostically – specific self-report scales. The scales and descriptions which follow are representative but by no means exhaustive of instruments that can be helpful in the primary care setting.

Broad-Based Screening Instruments

Broad-based self-report inventories, including both psychiatric symptoms as well as common physical complaints associated with mental health conditions, are an efficient method for initial screening. Some outpatient practices include a version of these scales as part of their standard new patient information and/or as part of annual updating of the patient's medical record. Patients are often asked to complete these checklists while in the waiting area or in the examination room awaiting their physician.

The General Health Questionnaire (*GHQ-12*; Goldberg & Williams, 1988) asks patients to rate the presence of a number of symptoms during the past several weeks. Items include "Have you recently been feeling unhappy and depressed? Have you recently lost sleep over worrying?" The GHQ has demonstrated moderate to high correlations with formal psychiatric diagnoses in primary care (Cano et al., 2001).

The *Symptom Checklist 10* (SCL-10; Derogatis, Lipman, & Covi, 1973) is a 10-item version derived from the longer SCL-90. The brief version includes six depressive items, two somatization questions, and two phobia/anxiety items. Respondents rate on a scale from 1 to 5 the extent to which these symptoms have been present during the past week. While the correlation with formal psychiatric diagnosis is a little lower than for the GHQ-12, the scale has good sensitivity and specificity – particularly for mood and anxiety disorders in primary care (Cano et al., 2001).

The *Primary Care Evaluation of Mental Disorders* (PRIME-MD; Spitzer et al., 1994) is more closely tied to the DSM system and includes two stages. Initially, patients complete a written inventory indicating whether any of 10 psychological and 15 somatic symptoms have been present within the past month. If scores are positive for specific clusters of items, a follow-up structured interview is conducted. The PRIME-MD is often used as a "gold standard" in primary care research. A complete self-report version without the interview, the Primary Health Questionnaire, may also be used for screening. Completed scales provide information about the extent to which patients meet criteria for one of the following: mood disorder, anxiety disorder, substance abuse, eating disorder, or somatoform disorder (Linton, 2004; Spitzer et al., 1994).

Anxiety Disorders
Generalized Anxiety Disorder
The *Generalized Anxiety Disorder Scale* includes six items assessing DSM-IV symptoms of generalized anxiety disorder. These include: feeling nervous or on edge; inability to control worrying; excessive worry; difficulty relaxing; difficulty with sitting still; being easily irritated; and feeling fearful that something bad might happen (Kroenke, Spitzer, Williams, Monahan, & Lowe, 2007). Patients rate themselves on a scale from 0 to 5. Total scores range from 0 to 21 with scores of 5 representing mild, 10 moderate, and 15 and above severe, anxiety symptoms. This scale, while focusing on generalized anxiety disorder, does appear to be reasonably sensitive to any current anxiety disorder diagnosis including panic disorder and social anxiety disorder (Kroenke et al., 2007).

Social Anxiety Disorder
Research suggests that the average age of onset for social anxiety disorder is 12 years. The *Screen for Child-Related Anxiety and Emotional Disorders* (*SCARED*) is a 41-item broad-based screen for anxiety disorders among pediatric patients. The seven-item SCARED social phobia subscale is completed by the parents. Representative items include "My child feels nervous with people he doesn't know well" and "My child is shy." "Each item is rated on 0–2 scale reflecting symptom frequency." Research suggests that parents of children with social anxiety disorder are more likely to validly report symptoms than the socially anxious child, themselves (Bailey, Chavira, Stein, & Stein, 2006).

Post Traumatic Stress Disorder (PTSD)

A four-item screening scale, the *Primary Care PTSD Screen*, was originally developed to screen combat veterans. The screen asks if the patient has ever had any frightening or upsetting experiences that, in the past month led to one of the following: (a) nightmares and flashbacks; (b) avoiding situations or avoiding thinking things that were reminders of the trauma; (c) constantly watchful or easily startled; and (d) feeling numb or detached from others or the immediate environment. The screen is considered "positive" if three of these items are answered in the affirmative (Prins et al., 2004).

Mood Disorders

Major Depressive Disorder

There are several commonly used self-report instruments for depressive symptoms that have been widely used in primary care. The original Beck Depression Inventory (BDI) is a 21-item self-report measure in which patients rate the relative severity of depressive symptoms (Beck & Steer, 1993). A revised version, the BDI-II reportedly can differentiate reactive and nonclinical sadness from a clinical mood disorder (Kush, 2001; Linton, 2004). A briefer, seven-item BDI has been developed specifically for primary care (BDI-PC; Beck, Steer, Ball, Ciervo, & Kabat, 1997). There has been concern, however, that the reduction in number of items weakens the scale's sensitivity (Linton, 2004).

The *Hamilton Depression Rating Scale* (Hamilton, 1967) has been used with medical patients as well as with patients in nursing home settings. The HAM-D is administered in a structured interview format and includes more emphasis on physical, neurovegetative symptoms. It is less efficient than the BDI because it is administered as an interview.

Finally, a scale specific to older patients is the *Geriatric Depression Scale (GDS)* (Linton, 2004; Yesavage et al., 1983). This instrument is also administered an interview style; however, responses are forced choice (yes/no) which can make it relatively efficient. The original GDS is 30 items, but there is a briefer 15-item version. It not only assesses mood, but also addresses interest in daily activities.

Bipolar Disorder

In recent years, there has been growing concern that bipolar mood disorder is being underdiagnosed. This is particularly true for bipolar II disorder in which major depressive symptoms alternate with those of hypomania. Hypomania is often not of sufficient severity to warrant psychiatric attention. As a result, it is more likely that patients with this condition will seek treatment during depressive episodes. A practical concern is that the pharmacotherapy-of-choice for major depressive disorder is not helpful by itself for bipolar disorder and may even worsen the condition. Therefore, it is important for primary care providers to be able to distinguish depressive episodes associated with bipolar II disorder from major depressive disorder.

The *Mood Disorder Questionnaire* (Hirschfeld et al., 2000) asks about the presence or absence of 13 symptoms of mania or hypomania including a need for markedly less sleep, racing thoughts, distractibility, excess spending, irritability, and excessive self-confidence. Patients are then asked whether several of these symptoms were concurrent. Finally, the respondent is asked about the extent of impairment associated with symptoms ranging from "no problem" to a "serious problem." Recent research with the instrument has found a sensitivity of .73 and specificity of .90 (Hirschfeld et al., 2000).

There is increasing evidence that bipolar disorder may have its onset prior to or in early adolescence. Connors has developed a 10-item parent rating scale (the *Connors Abbreviated Parent Questionnaire*) for early onset bipolar disorder. The items are somewhat different than those for adults and include symptoms such as crying easily and often; temper outbursts and explosions; disturbing other children; and having a short attention span. The scale also appears to be comparably sensitive and specific as the adult scale mentioned above even though the items reflect symptoms distinctive for pediatric bipolar disorder (Tillman & Geller, 2005). Of note, despite the comorbidity and similarity of ADHD and bipolar symptoms in children, the scale was able to differentiate these two conditions (Tillman & Geller, 2005).

Substance Abuse

Alcohol Abuse and Dependence

There are several alcohol questionnaires that have been widely used in primary care. The **CAGE** questionnaire is a four-item screen that is typically conducted as part of the clinical interview. Patients are asked: (1) "Have you tried to **C**ut down on your drinking?"; (2) "Have others been **A**nnoyed with you because of your drinking?"; (3) "Have you felt **G**uilty because of your drinking?"; (4) "Have you had a morning **E**ye opener?" A positive response to one of these questions suggests a possible alcohol problem while two positive responses suggest a probable alcohol problem (Mayfield, McCleod, & Hall, 1974).

The *Alcohol Use Disorders Identification Test* (AUDIT; Allen, Reinert, & Volk, 2001) is a 10-item rating scale which includes social consequences of drinking as well as frequency of alcohol use and quantity consumed in a drinking episode. An item on binge drinking (six or more drinks on a given occasion) is also included. The scale was originally developed by the World Health Organization and has been normed in at least six different countries (Linton, 2004). The scale can be administered as a pencil-and-paper measure or as a brief interview. Since it assesses a broader continuum of drinking behavior, the AUDIT is particularly useful for detecting earlier stages of problem alcohol use.

The *Michigan Alcohol Screening Test* (MAST; Selzer, 1971) focuses more on social consequences of heavy drinking. Items include blackouts and alcohol-related legal problems. A briefer version, the S-MAST, includes an item asking if the respondent has ever attended a meeting of Alcoholics Anonymous. Recent research suggests that this question yields a number of false positives. The MAST also does not differentiate between past and present alcohol-related problems. Additionally, because it covers a broad range of social dysfunction, a positive score is usually indicative of a problem. However the problem may not necessarily be alcohol abuse. Thus, while the MAST has reasonable sensitivity, specificity has been a significant concern (Chang, Goetz, Wilkins-Haug, & Berman, 1999).

The *TWEAK* appears to have particular promise with female patients and has been used to screen for alcohol use in pregnant women. TWEAK is an acronym: T – tolerance "How many drinks does it take before you feel the first effects of alcohol?" or "How many drinks does it take before the effects of alcohol make you fall asleep or pass out?"; W – worried "Have your friends or relatives worried about your drinking in the past year?"; E – eye opener "Do you sometimes take a drink in the morning before you get up?"; A – amnesia "Are there times when you drink and afterwards can't remember what you said or did?"; K/C – cut down "Do you sometimes feel the need to cut down on your drinking?" (Russell, 1994). The TWEAK question about tolerance was designed to detect at risk drinking – specifically among pregnant women (Mengel, Searight, & Cook, 2006). The TWEAK does appear to have greater specificity among women than the CAGE or the MAST (Mengel et al., 2006).

Alcohol Withdrawal: A common issue arising in the emergency department, as well as on medical-surgical inpatient units, is the evaluation of patients who may be withdrawing from alcohol. Often, these patients are admitted to the hospital following an accident or because of an acute illness. Their pattern of alcohol use may not become known until approximately 6–8 hours after the patient's last drink when they began to show withdrawal symptoms such as tremulousness. The *Clinical Institute Withdrawal Assessment for Alcohol – Revised* (CIWA-Ar) is a 10-item rating scale in which nine common alcohol withdrawal symptoms are rated on a 0–7 scale with respect to severity and a tenth dimension, orientation to time, rated on a 0–4 scale. The nine dimensions are nausea/vomiting, tremors, anxiety, agitation, paroxysmal sweats, tactile disturbances, auditory disturbances, visual disturbances, and headache. The total points are added and the patient is placed into one of three categories of alcohol withdrawal: absent to minimal; mild to moderate; and severe (Sullivan, Sykora, Schneiderman, Naranjo, & Sellers, 1989). Generally speaking, patients with mild to moderate and above levels of withdrawal are given anxiolytic medication until symptoms subside. The objective of the CIWA is to detect and quantify alcohol withdrawal so that more severe outcomes such as seizures and even death can be prevented (Reoux & Miller, 2000).

Cigarettes

The *Fagerstrom Tolerance Questionnaire* is an eight-item self-report instrument helpful in assessing the patient's level of smoking (Heatherton, Kozlowski, Frecker, & Fagerstrom, 1991). The scale focuses on the level of physical dependency on cigarettes based on several factors: (a) time to first cigarette of the day upon awakening; (b) number of cigarettes smoked per day; (c) early morning smoking; (d) managing refraining from smoking in prohibited areas; (e) smoking when ill; and (f) level of nicotine in current cigarette brand. As an added question, clinicians may ask the patient to choose which daily cigarette would be most difficult to give up. Scores range from 0 to 11 with higher scores indicating a significant dependence on tobacco. The time elapsed from waking to first cigarette is a particularly meaningful index of nicotine dependence. The scale can be particularly helpful in determining whether a patient would benefit from nicotine replacement therapy and/or other pharmacotherapy such as buproprion (Zyban) or varenicline (Chantix) for smoking cessation.

Other Drugs of Abuse

The World Health Organization has developed a broader primary care screening measure to assess for drug abuse as well as alcohol. The *Alcohol, Smoking, and Substance Involve-*

ment Screening Test is an eight-item instrument requiring less than 5 minutes to complete (Connors & Stewart, 2004).

The *Drug Abuse Screening Test* (Skinner, 1982) is a 20-item questionnaire focusing upon social and physical consequences of drug use (Connors & Stewart, 2004).

Dementia

The *Mini Mental Status Examination* (MMSE; Folstein, Folstein, & McHugh, 1975) is a brief, efficient, and standardized method for assessing cognitive functioning. It is primarily used to assess older patients when there is concern about the possibility of dementia. The scale has been translated into multiple languages and also has well-developed norms and cutoff scores. Domains assessed include orientation to place and time, attention, concentration, language comprehension and repetition, written expression, and visual-spatial skills. With a maximum score of 30, a score of 24 has typically been used as a cutoff for indicating the presence of cognitive impairment. However, it is important to use age and education-based norms when assessing patients. For example, someone with a sixth grade education obtaining a score of 19 would be at the 25th percentile for their level of education. While the global score is well below the cutoff, the corresponding percentile does not indicate clinically significant impairment (Crum et al., 1993).

The *Clock Drawing Test* involves presenting the patient with a predrawn circle and asking them to draw the hands and numbers for a clock set at a specific time (e.g., 10 minutes before 11) and appears to be a very sensitive task. Clock drawing involves recall, verbal comprehension, as well as sequencing and visual-spatial relationships. There are multiple formal scoring systems for the task (Freedman et al., 1994). Many, if not most clinicians analyze the clock qualitatively. Dimensions to consider include the placement of numbers, the sequence of numbers, the distinction between minute and hour hands as well as whether they reflect the time requested and finally, accurate proportional distribution of both hands and the numbers on the clock face. The clock test does appear to be sensitive to early stages of dementia – often indicating the condition well before any markers would appear on an imaging study (Searight, 1999).

Attention Deficit/Hyperactivity Disorder (ADHD)

Children

There are a variety of behavioral rating scales for use in assessing disruptive behavior disorders including oppositional defiant, ADHD, and conduct disorders. These instruments include the *Connors Rating Scale*, the *Child Behavior Checklist,* and the *Vanderbilt Scale.* Many of these instruments reflect the 18 DSM symptoms of ADHD and ask the respondent – either the parent or teacher – to rate the frequency with which these behaviors occur. In addition to assessing for ADHD symptoms, the Vanderbilt Scale also includes items addressing conduct disorder, oppositional defiant disorder, and anxiety and mood disorders. The respondent is also asked to provide ratings about the extent to which symptoms are impairing day-to-day activity. There are two versions of the scale – one for parents and one for teachers. The Vanderbilt is part of the American Academy of Pediatrics toolkit for ADHD.

Adults

As clinicians have become more aware of the chronic nature of ADHD, several scales have been developed to assess symptoms in adults. These scales, as a general rule, attempt to capture adult-specific versions of symptoms. For example, rather than the childhood behavior of running around the room and having difficulty with remaining seated, a sense of inner restlessness might better capture hyperactivity in adults. The adult-specific ADHD scales include a version of the *Connors*, the *Brown ADD Scales* as well as the *Copeland Scale*. An instrument developed specifically for evaluating these adult symptoms in primary care is the *Adult Self-Report Scale – VI.1 Screener* (ASRS-VI.I). This six-item tool asks about the frequency, on a 0–5 scale, of symptoms including difficulty remembering appointments, postponing tasks that are cognitively demanding, and poor organizational skills (World Health Organization, 2003).

Clinical Application of Screening Instruments in Primary Care

While the idea of using patient self-report instruments or very brief yes-no types of structured questions may be particularly attractive given primary care's time constraints, these instruments should never be used in isolation for diagnosis. Most psychiatric tools, when applied to primary care patients, have reasonably good sensitivity but are often nonspecific. Psychologists are typically well-educated in use of these types of tools and know that any type of psychological testing should be used for diagnosis and treatment planning only in conjunction with a thorough history and interview. This guideline is particularly true in primary care where time pressures could lead to over-reliance on paper-and-pencil instruments. In using measures like those listed above, a general rule of thumb is that a clinically elevated score usually indicates some type of psychiatric condition. However, establishing that condition with any precision requires follow-up interviewing.

An overarching problem in using psychiatric rating scales in the medical setting is that many of the symptoms of mental health conditions are physical, nonspecific, and may be caused by a range of medical and/or mental health conditions. In assessing patients for major depressive disorder, it is important to remember that a number of the core symptoms, such as sleep disturbance, appetite and weight change, diminished energy, and problems with concentration and attention may arise from medical conditions, medications, and/or hospitalization. Coyne, Thompson, Palmer, and Kagee (2000) found that in applying depression screens to primary care patients, the customary practice of totaling the number of symptoms and their relative severity and then classifying patients into depressed or non-depressed groups was questionably valid. Depression was likely to be overdiagnosed because of the overlap between depression's vegetative symptoms and symptoms of many medical conditions. The presence of dysphoric mood and/or anhedonia were key symptoms discriminating depressed from nondepressed patients in this setting. However, at the same time, it is important that primary care providers remain alert to the possibility of severe major depressive disorder. Research suggests that on the average, about 45%

of people who effect suicide have contacted their primary care physicians in the month prior to their death (Ruddy et al., 2008).

A Caveat: The Risks of Epidemiological Reasoning in Primary Care

A central problem with epidemiological reasoning in primary care is that most of the conditions that physicians in this setting address are self-limiting – meaning that most complaints resolve on their own. Medical advice (e.g., rest and fluids) and/or a prescription may expedite this process and improve patient comfort. Occasionally, however, one of these usually benign symptoms signals a life-threatening condition. One of the major challenges of primary care medicine is to stay alert to this possibility. Groopman (2007) in his discussion with pediatrician, Victoria Rogers McEvoy, uses this analogy:

> Imagine watching a train go by. You are looking for one face in the window. Car after car passes. If you become distracted or inattentive, you risk missing the person or, if the train picks up too much speed, the faces begin to blur and you can't see the one you're seeking. "That's what primary care medicine is like.". . . It's much harder than the proverbial needle in a haystack, because the haystack is not moving. Each day there is a steady flow of patients before your eyes. You're doing well baby checks, examinations for school, making sure each one is up to date on his vaccinations. It can become rote, and you stop observing closely. Then you have the endless number of kids who are cranky and have a fever, and it's almost always a virus or strep throat. They can all blur. But then there is that one time it's meningitis (p. 77).

The possibility of missing a life-threatening condition is the often unstated danger in thinking epidemiologically. Low probability events do happen. Ignoring the possibility that what appeared to be a benign symptom of a self-limiting condition actually indicates a serious life-threatening illness, is a crucial mistake that all practicing physicians fear. In primary care, this is particularly problematic since most presenting complaints are not associated with serious or life-threatening illness.

When seeing patients as part of this assessment process, psychologists, while not expected to diagnose nonpsychiatric conditions, should be able to recognize when aspect(s) of a patient's history, symptoms, and/or demographics are not generally consistent with a mental health condition. For example, weight loss, while a symptom of major depressive disorder, should be suspect in the absence of unchanged eating patterns. Similarly, chest pain, even when no medical etiology is initially determined, while often a symptom of panic disorder, should trigger the psychologist to consider a nonpsychiatric etiology – particularly when the discomfort lasts more than an hour in duration. Medical students and residents, when presenting a new patient's symptoms to a supervising physician, are often asked "What's the worst thing this could be?" (Groopman, 2007). Primary care psychologists should consider this question as well.

The Use of Psychological Interventions in Primary Care

Since the number of patients with behavioral and psychiatric issues far exceeds those presenting in mental health settings (Robinson, 2005), traditional individual psychotherapy would have minimal coverage and impact in primary care. With its population-oriented approach, primary care mental health is symptom focused and also relies on patient self-management and educational intervention strategies. As a result, the present-day primary care psychologist will draw upon a heterogeneous group of intervention strategies ranging from computer-guided counseling to 5-minute protocol interventions for alcohol abuse to 15- to 30-minute highly structured counseling sessions for less-specific psychosocial problem. Evidence for some of these approaches – particularly briefer educationally oriented interventions for alcohol, smoking, and exercise – does support their effectiveness. As interventions become less focused and specific, evidence for their efficacy in primary care becomes more limited. This is an area that warrants future research directed toward development of a set of evidence-based guidelines for the primary care psychologist.

The Economic Benefits of Population-Based Primary Care Psychology: The Problem of High Utilizers

At a population level, one of the significant factors associated with increased health care costs are high utilizers of medical care. Multiple studies have found that in large managed care plans, somewhere between 10% and 15% of patients may use approximately 60–70% of the plan's medical services. An early high utilizer study concluded that 60% of all physician office visits were with one of two groups of patients: patients expressing psychosocial stress somatically or those with chronic illness exacerbated by stress (Seaburn, Lorenz, Gunn, Gawinski, & Mauksch, 1996). High utilizers are frequently patients with a number of nonspecific somatic complaints or medically unexplained illnesses such as irritable bowel syndrome (IBS) or chronic fatigue syndrome (Johnson, 2008). For example, patients with IBS, a nonspecific GI condition strongly associated with anxiety and depressive symptoms, enrolled in health maintenance organization (HMO) were significantly more likely to undergo gallbladder surgery, appendectomies, hysterectomies and back surgery. Overall, IBS is associated with annual direct medical costs of 8 billion dollars (Johnson, 2008). Both major and minor depressive illness are associated with increased utilization for nonpsychiatric medical conditions as well (Beekman, Deeg, Braaam, Smit, & Van Tilberg, 1997).

There is some evidence from research on collaborative care programs that the addition of psychological services may reduce inappropriate medical utilization. A large study conducted in Hawaii found that targeted mental health interventions of the type described in the remainder of this book saved an average of $350 per patient compared to those patients seen in traditional medical settings who actually had increased costs of $750 per patient. Much of the benefit of cost offset comes in the form of reduced hospital days (Cummings, O'Donohue, Hayes, & Follette, 2001). In an economic analysis of the top 10 primary care complaints, the cost of evaluating nonspecific chest pain was over $21,000, while the cost of establishing an organic cause for the symptom was approximately $1,400 (Cummings et al., 2001; Kroenke & Mangelsdorf, 1989). The significantly higher cost of evaluating nonspecific pain stems from the fact that since a cause cannot be readily determined, the patient receives a much greater number of diagnostic tests. Cost offset appears to be most pronounced for three subgroups of patients: primary care patients with multiple vague (medically unexplained) complaints, acutely ill hospitalized elderly patients, and nonelderly adults with alcohol problems (Bray, Frank, McDaniel, & Heldring, 2004).

In a traditional fee-for-service system, collaborative care, while good for patients, has few economic advantages for health care organizations and providers. However, in capitated plans, where a health care group is paid a yearly retainer to manage a specific panel of patients, the value of available psychological consultation can be considerable. Other organizations in which psychological consultation should demonstrate some economic benefits are in the Veterans Administration system which is now adding primary care psychology as part of their outpatient services. Including primary care psychologists in disease management programs such as those developed by Medicaid and Medicare for patients with conditions such as asthma, chronic obstructive pulmonary disease, and diabetes would also likely show significant cost savings.

A Little Can Mean a Lot: Population-Based Impact of Weight Loss

In examining interventions from an epidemiological perspective, the focus is not on individual-level cure but instead on larger-scale harm reduction. Given that a particular primary care physician may have a patient base of multiple thousand, risk reductions of a small magnitude can yield significant benefits in a particular patient cohort. For example, a prevalence study of obesity among Michigan family practice patients found rates to be significantly higher than in the state's general population. In this large pool of primary care patients, the age-adjusted rate of being overweight was 53% with 27.5% of patients classified as being severely overweight. These figures are significantly higher than national studies of obesity indicating a prevalence of overweight at 33% and severely overweight at 14% (Noel, Hickner, Ettenhofer, & Gauthier, 1998). Given the morbidity burden associated with obesity, it is understandable that primary care patients would be more likely to be overweight. From a harm reduction perspective, even a modest weight loss of about 15 pounds per person will significantly reduce the prevalence of overweight and obesity. For example, in the Michigan patient pool, a 15-pound reduction reduced the prevalence of overweight from 53% to 38% and for those severely overweight from 28% to 18%. A focus on limited and realistic weight loss reduction is likely to have broader population-based impact than a narrower focus on selected patients with substantial weight problems. This pattern carries over to weight-related health risks. Even though weight loss may not be great enough to bring someone below the BMI cutoff for being overweight, even modest weight reductions of 5–10% reduce the risk for type II diabetes and cardiovascular disease.

Examples of Brief Intervention in Primary Care

Brief Feedback and Harm Reduction for Alcohol Abuse

Reducing alcohol use has been the focus of a number of good quality studies of the effectiveness of brief interventions in primary care. Research typically focuses on a comparison of treatment as usual versus one or more specific interventions to reduce alcohol consumption. In addressing alcohol use, reduced consumption may have benefits that are not directly due to physiological effects of alcohol. Accidental deaths, one of the leading causes of death among young adults, are associated with increased alcohol consumption. If alcohol use is reduced from five standard drinks per day to two standard drinks per day the relative risk of dying decreases by a factor of five.

Brief interventions studied have ranged from ultra-brief (5 minutes or less) to brief (a one-time 10- to 15-minute episode of counseling) to extended brief (several 10- to 15-minute sessions) treatment. Ultra-brief counseling of 5 minutes or less involves asking about the patient's recent alcohol consumption, providing brief advice about reasonable drinking, and a corresponding recommendation to reduce intake but without providing any specific strategies. At the next level are interventions with a duration of approximately 10–15 minutes and include assessment, advice, and strategies to reduce alcohol consumption. Typically this counseling is conducted in one session with the possibility of 3- to 5-minute boosters being offered in subsequent office visits. Finally, extended brief intervention typically includes several office visits with 10- to 15-minute sessions in which ongoing assessment of alcohol use is conducted with corresponding advice and behavior modification. These visits typically occur over multiple months (Ballesteros, Gonzalez-Pinto, Querejeta, & Arino, 2004).

The interventions themselves vary somewhat. Several techniques demonstrating effectiveness as brief interventions include the five "A"s (Ask, Advise, Assess, . . .) and FRAMES, structured protocols discussed in the next chapter. However, shared aspects of brief interventions include feedback using self-report information about alcohol consumption, such as the CAGE, or physiological indicators such as blood pressure to increase patient awareness of the adverse effects of drinking. The second component, direct advice, usually focuses on high-risk situations for alcohol consumption and developing strategies to reduce alcohol use. Finally, the provider works collaboratively with the patient in goal setting for reduced alcohol consumption (O'Connor & Whaley, 2007).

Research has shown that ultra-brief interventions, consisting of one 5-minute physician counseling session, significantly decrease self-reported alcohol consumption while a 10- to 15-minute session has been associated with reduced drinking validated by laboratory GGT (liver function) levels. Additionally, this brief intervention has been associated with reduced blood pressure, lowered triglyceride levels, and fewer sick days. Fleming and colleagues developed Project TREAT, a structured primary care intervention involving physician consultation every 3 months and monthly gamma-glutamyl-transferase (GGT; a liver enzyme) (liver function). levels. A 5-year follow-up found that those patients in the program had fewer hospital days, sick days, and lower mortality (Fleming et al., 1998).

Brief Alcohol Counseling Reduces Fetal Mortality

Among patients who are not yet alcohol dependent, a variety of brief interventions appear to be helpful in reducing drinking. Research suggests that 10–30% of patients will reduce drinking as a result of these brief interventions. One particular subgroup of problem drinkers are pregnant women. Alcohol consumption during pregnancy is associated with both fetal alcohol syndrome (FAS) as well as fetal alcohol effects in which the cognitive difficulties are present without the FAS physical features. In a study of pregnant women randomly assigned to brief primary care counseling intervention versus those receiving standard care, there were pronounced differences in fetal mortality. Estimated fetal mortality in the intervention group was estimated to be 9/1000 compared with 29/1000 in the assessment alone condition. This is a substantial reduction when compared with general population fetal mortality rates of 11.02 for Black, non-Hispanic and 5.57 for Hispanic women (O'Connor & Whaley, 2007). Providing brief intervention or assessment earlier in the course of pregnancy was associated with greater likelihood of reduced alcohol consumption (O'Connor & Whaley, 2007). Of interest, even personalized written materials emphasizing assessment feedback, without face-to-face contact, reduced binge drinking by 10% among these women. Pregnancy is often a significant impetus to eliminate or reduce cigarette and alcohol use.

Brief Intervention: Results of Meta-Analyses and Comparative Outcomes

Results of a meta-analysis indicated effect sizes for individual studies of brief alcohol intervention ranging from −.05 to −.51 with an average effect of −.26 (Ballesteros et al., 2004). This small to moderate, yet robust, effect size suggests that relatively brief, yet targeted, counseling can reduce health risk behavior. Another meta-analysis found that among heavy drinkers, brief intervention reduced alcohol consumption twofold as compared with a no intervention group (Wilk, Jensen, & Havighurst, 1997). It is important to recognize that effective brief intervention does not usually lead to cessation of alcohol use but a reduction in quantity, and possibly, frequency (i.e., drinking days) of consumption. Some studies have found that ultra-brief and more extensive brief interventions are equally effective (Aalto et al., 2000). The results of the limited number of brief intervention studies targeted to pregnant women currently consuming alcohol suggests that factors such as pregnancy may increase amenability to intervention.

Psychotherapy Without a Therapist: Online, Self-Paced Treatment

Another approach requiring minimal provider time and resources is online psychotherapy. MoodGYM, an online intervention for depression, features a set of modules intended to be completed in a specific sequence (Christensen, Griffiths, Mackinnon, & Brittliffe, 2006). MoodGYM is a free, open access website. The modules include an assessment of symptoms using the Goldberg Depression and Anxiety Scales (Goldberg, Bridges, Duncan-Jones, & Grayson, 1988), feedback on the assessment using six fictional characters, a description of basic cognitive-behavioral concepts, and an orientation to the worksheets and online workbook. The second module focuses on distorted cognitions and helps participants identify, effectively challenge, and alter these thought patterns. In the third module, behavioral strategies to address unpleasant affect are presented. The Pleasant Events Schedule is employed to increase both physical and social activity. Module four addresses stressors and stress management and includes assessment of sources of life stress, coping strategies for interpersonal stressors, and downloadable audio relaxation recordings. The final module describes problem-solving skills for relationships as well as information about common comorbid conditions with depression.

In attempting to isolate active components of MoodGYM, Christensen et al. (2006) found that the second module, focusing on identifying and refuting distorted cognitions, was most strongly associated with improvement. However, despite an estimated 50% of the total participants meeting criteria for clinical depression, at least 70% of those completing the assessment failed to complete even one treatment module. While meta-analyses of typical outpatient cognitive-behavioral therapy have yielded effect sizes in the .8–1.0 range, the estimated effect size for the effective intervention components from Mood GYM was .4. It is likely that some type of monitoring system would have increased the numbers of individuals completing the intervention as well as improved MOOD-GYM's effectiveness. Other studies have found e-mails and/or phone calls improve participation with an online intervention (Tate, Jackvony, & Wing, 2003). Online psychoeducational treatment has considerable promise for efficient, cost-effective treatment having population wide impact. Research to date does suggest that individuals who seek out websites with these modules are experiencing psychiatric distress.

Counseling and Psychotherapy in Primary Care

While limited by methodological issues, research on primary care interventions does indicate that they are effective. Focusing primarily on interventions provided in Britain's National Health Service (NHS) system, Bower, Rowland, and Hardy (2003) found a significant, yet modest, effect size for brief counseling compared with usual medical care. The primary care interventions varied from well-described cognitive-behavioral therapy to psychodynamic therapy to person-centered treatment to "generic" counseling. When available diagnoses were reviewed, most patients appeared to have symptoms of anxiety and depression or less-specific emotional difficulties lasting for less than 6 months duration (Bower et al., 2003).

Further caveats include suggestions that primary care patients may exhibit lower levels of psychiatric symptoms than patients seen in the specialty mental health sector. There was also concern about the durability and magnitude of primary care counseling benefits. While a statistically significant level of improvement was obtained by those receiving counseling versus those receiving usual care, only about one third of those receiving counseling moved from the clinically distressed to nondistressed range. The differences in psychiatric symptoms between those receiving counseling and those in the physician-only typical care group were not maintained beyond 6 months (Bower et al., 2003). In the NHS, patients were generally satisfied with counseling received and some types of health care utilization were lower in this group. However, overall health costs were not significantly reduced among those patients receiving counseling (Bower & Rowland, 2006).

The British data stand in marked contrast to the US studies on high utilizers and patients with somatoform disorders. The provision of counseling in the National Health Service in which counselors and psychiatric social workers are colocated in general medical practices has a much longer history in Britain than in the United States. The lack of specificity about the types of approaches being used with primary care patients makes it difficult to interpret the British findings. However, review of case reports and practice literature from the NHS suggest that a broader, less symptom-focused approach, influenced by psychodynamic theory, is common (Balint, 1964).

Stepped Care: A Model for Resource Efficient Treatment

Stepped care is a resource-efficient approach that is consistent with how primary care physicians approach patient care. As noted in Chapters 1 and 2, primary care physicians are the first point of contact for patients and are trained to treat a broad range of presenting problems. If an initial approach to treatment such as "conservative therapy" for lower back musculoskeletal pain is not associated with improvement in 10–14 days, a second tier intervention might be to refer the patient for physical therapy. If antiinflammatory medication together with regular physical therapy and back exercises that the patient carries out on their own are ineffective, a referral to an orthopedic specialist may be the third step.

The general approach in primary care is to address problems with the least intrusive and invasive methods first and then to gradually add treatments and if the patient still is not responsive or only partially responsive, to refer them to a specialist. While this model is certainly not used with all patients and there are patients who are referred directly to specialists, this approach is very consistent with the philosophy of primary care. The majority of patients will benefit from levels 1 and 2 interventions leaving a minority to be referred. The physician diagnoses and treats most patients that they see – only turning to referrals for surgeons and other specialists when an initial treatment and/or possibly a second intervention (often added to the first) does not result in significant improvement. As noted in Chapter 2, given that the majority of patients seen in primary care have nonlife-threatening conditions, less intensive – "conservative" – treatments are likely to be effective a good deal of the time.

Conceptually, stepped care includes the following three key features:

1. The initial treatment of choice is the least intrusive and disruptive to the patient's ongoing lifestyle.
2. Treatment resources are used with optimal efficiency – typically the minimum treatment established to produce therapeutic change.
3. In the provider's judgment, the treatment has a reasonable probability of being effective with a particular patient – in the context of their illness and life circumstances (Berner et al., 2008; Sobell & Sobell, 2000).

As an example, a stepped approach for psychological treatment of Obsessive-Compulsive Disorder (OCD) may begin with bibliotherapy. For those patients demonstrating a minimal response to bibliotherapy, brief education may be added. If symptoms persist, cognitive-behavioral therapy may be the third step. Tolin, Diefenbach, Maltby, and Hannan (2005) found that 20% of a group of patients with OCD responded to Step 1 and 30% to Step 2. Of the remaining 50%, nearly three-quarters demonstrated significant symptom improvement with cognitive-behavioral therapy (Tolin et al., 2005). A possible fourth step for the remaining 25% would be to add a psychotropic medication such as a selective serotonin reuptake inhibitor (SSRI).

A stepped care algorithm for managing depression in primary care is regularly used by the author. For patients with an acute onset of symptoms with no prior history of major depressive disorder, 60–70% should demonstrate significant improvement with SSRI pharmacotherapy alone. For patients with a longer-standing history of major depressive disorder, a significant family history of the condition, early adult onset, and/or a comorbid psychiatric disorder, cognitive therapy such as problem-solving therapy (see Chapter 8) may be a useful addition. Research suggests that the addition of cognitive-behavioral therapy also reduces the risk of relapse. When this combination is ineffective, third-line treatment may include adding a second psychotropic agent such as a stimulant. Among depressed female patients in a conflictual relationship – a fairly common pairing – marital or family therapy is adjunctive treatment. This latter intervention is associated with better outcome among patients with MDD in distressed relationships and is associated with decreased likelihood of a recurrence of depression (Hooley & Teasdale, 1989; Jacobson, Dobson, Fruzzetti, Schmaling, & Salusky, 1991).

In the absence of data to guide decisions about moving from one level to the next, clinicians rely on their own judgment and heuristics derived from previous treatment episodes. While formal stepped care algorithms appear logical and efficient, they are governed by evidence-based protocols – the majority of which were developed on patients with a specific diagnosis without additional psychiatric or medical conditions (fibromyalgia, hypertension, and generalized anxiety disorder) or psychosocial complications (e.g., poverty and lack of transportation). This is a fertile area for applied research – particularly in the primary care arena where stepped care needs to include attention to the comorbidity of psychiatric and medical conditions. Examples include type II diabetes and obesity in a patient with schizophrenia or the common combination of opioid dependence, major depressive disorder, and chronic low back pain.

Again, there may be situations in which a primary care provider would bypass levels one and two. There is some evidence that educationally focused interventions in primary care, often delivered by nursing staff, may be effective with relatively recent onset eating disorders (Palmer, Birchall, McGrain, & Sullivan, 2002). However, for patients who have medical complications such as electrolyte imbalances or who have lost substantial amounts of weight, in which delay could be life threatening, appropriate clinical care would be to go directly to a level III specialized intervention. Similarly, a depressed patient with pronounced suicidal thinking or psychotic symptoms should usually be directly referred to a psychiatrist, a level III intervention.

Conclusion

The principal objective of this chapter has been to encourage psychologists to approach clinical problems from a population-based perspective. Knowledge of epidemiology in terms of risk factors and comorbidities, as well as demographic patterns, can be very helpful in conducting efficient assessments. Psychologists should also recognize that levels of psychiatric distress are likely to be much higher in primary care than in the general population but at the same time are often comorbid with many chronic medical conditions. Psychologists who are attuned to these medical comorbidities can be extremely helpful in addressing issues such as depression which is associated with nonadherence and deterioration in health status of patients with illnesses such as diabetes or hypertension. As noted in Chapters 2 and 3, it is critical that mental health professionals without formal medical training maintain appropriate respect for medical illnesses. In using psychological screening instruments, clinicians should remember that many of the nonspecific symptoms of mental health conditions can also indicate a nonpsychiatric medical condition. While psychologists are not expected to diagnose outside of their area of professional expertise, they should maintain awareness of clinical features that are not consistent with psychiatric illness when conducting evaluations. Finally, intervening from an epidemiological perspective involves providing the minimal level of care that is likely to be effective. This stepped care approach is necessary to reach the broadest number of patients as well as to conserve resources including time, money, and patient cooperation.

Chapter 5

Brief Counseling for Health Risk Behaviors

The Five "A"s and FRAMES

While many psychologists may believe that assessment and intervention with health risk behavior requires, at minimum, several hour long office visits, research reviewed in the previous chapter indicates brief assessment and advice can have considerable impact. This chapter reviews two models, the five "A"s and FRAMES, developed specifically for primary care physicians. These protocols are time efficient and have demonstrated efficacy in reducing smoking and alcohol consumption, as well as in increasing physical activity levels.

The Five "A"s

The five "A"s (Ask, Advise, Assess, Assist, and Arrange) are an efficient strategy for addressing risk behavior such as smoking and drinking and may be adapted to dietary adherence and regular exercise. More recently, this framework has been used to address psychiatric problems in primary care as well (Hunter, Goodie, Oordt, & Dobmeyer, 2009). This approach is becoming better known in primary care because of its use as part of a national effort at reducing smoking during pregnancy (Fiore et al., 2000). The five "A"s are a framework in which the individual dimensions are adapted to the type, severity, and duration of the problem being addressed (Hunter et al., 2009). Each of these dimensions will be discussed in detail.

Ask

Several dimensions are helpful to consider when asking about health risk behavior. First, in primary care, excessive alcohol use, smoking, or a sedentary lifestyle are rarely presenting problems. Instead, the effects of these behaviors such as chronic GI distress, insomnia, chronic cough, or fatigue will be chief complaints. Questions are often asked presumptively so as to obtain more valid information. Rather than asking "Do you drink alcohol?", a more accurate picture of alcohol use is likely to be obtained with the question, "How often have you had an alcoholic drink in the past month?" There are suggestions that paper-and-pencil self-report inventories may yield more valid information about health risk behavior than direct interview questions (for examples of brief self-report inventories, see Chapter 4). Standard dimensions to consider include frequency, duration and in cases of substance use, quantity.

Asking also overlaps into assessment – particularly when evaluating the patient's willingness to alter this behavior: "During the past 6 months have you attempted to diet or otherwise change your eating habits?" The assessment may also include attention to factors that are barriers to change. For heavy drinking, if patients regularly go to the tavern immediately after work and if the social network in the workplace is composed primarily of fellow drinkers, assessing the importance and impact of this interpersonal network will be particularly important.

The Health Beliefs Model (Champion & Skinner, 2008) includes attention to the patient's perceived susceptibility to an adverse health outcome. While asking questions such as "What effects do you think smoking will have for you in the future?" are often helpful in determining whether the patient is realistically appraising risks, these should be used with some caution. Research suggests that patients engaging in behavior such as smoking underestimate the extent to which regular cigarette use results in long-term harm. For most health risk behaviors, barriers to change actually appear to be more significant in maintaining risk behavior than perceived susceptibility to harm, perceived severity of a negative outcome, and perceived benefits of change (Champion & Skinner, 2008).

Advise

A key element in advising patients is being able to link behavior change to the patient's unique, personal health status. For patients who are regular marijuana users, linking the frequent episodes of illness such as colds and respiratory problems as well as the financial cost of smoking cannabis, can have considerable impact. One of the most commonly used health indicators of excess alcohol use in primary care is blood pressure. When making this linkage, defensiveness is less likely to be aroused if statements are made in the third person and in an emotionally neutral manner rather than a more threatening, first or second person "you" statement. A defensive reaction is less likely if the provider begins with an "I" ("I recommend that you. . .") rather than a "You" ("You need to. . .") statement. For example, "I see that your blood pressure is higher today than is normal for someone your age. Drinking alcohol frequently has been found to be associated with increasing blood pressure, I recommend that you stop or reduce how much alcohol you drink." rather than "Your blood pressure today is very high. If you keep drinking heavily it is simply going to get worse. You need to stop drinking."

The next aspect of this stage is to address the patient's openness to solutions. After the risk of continuing smoking or drinking is addressed, useful follow-up questions are:

"Is this something you are concerned about?"; "Are you interested in making this change in the next 30 days?" If the patient responds that they are, the next step is to describe one or more strategies to assist them with change. For smokers, these may include a nicotine patch, pharmacotherapy such as bupropion, referral for behaviorally oriented stimulus control strategies, and/or a smoking cessation support group. While educational handouts are helpful for reinforcing recommendations and framing treatment options, printed material should not be used in place of direct discussion. In either the "Advise" or "Assess" phase, psychologists may encounter resistance or significant ambivalence surrounding lifestyle change. Patients exhibiting these reactions often are unresponsive to direct suggestion and may instead, benefit from further assessment of motivational factors such as their stage of change (Chapter 6) or their values (Chapter 7).

Agree

This phase focuses on establishing an agreement about the specific plan for change. A collaborative approach increases patient ownership and, in turn, is more likely to be carried out. Patients should be encouraged to choose change strategies that best fit their lifestyle. If the patient appears hesitant, they should also be encouraged to indicate if none of the options are acceptable to them. If this is the case, it is helpful to ask the patient directly what strategies they believe will be helpful to them. Importantly, patients should be asked these questions in a spirit of curiosity and collaboration. In addition, if the patient has been successful in other health arenas (such as quitting smoking but now wants to stop drinking), the provider can highlight the prior success and use it as a foundation of skills for addressing current health risk behavior; "You were able to stop smoking on your own. What did you do to succeed in quitting smoking that you think might work for cutting back on alcohol?"

Assist

The chief focus here is to help the patient with implementing their plan for change. It is particularly important that the plan is consistent with the patient's lifestyle. For example, for a patient who has been sedentary for several years, beginning a daily 30-minute jogging program is unrealistic and likely to fail. An initial intervention might be to walk or jog in place for 5–10 minutes each day while watching television and then for the next week, adding another 5 minutes of activity per day. Week three may include walking around the block for 15 minutes. Implementation will include problem solving to address environmental or social barriers that arise in choosing a strategy that can be realistically implemented.

   If the patient does seem ambivalent about initiating change and/or cites multiple barriers, it is often useful to return to a discussion of the patient's level of motivation for change with questions such as "How important is it for you to reduce your drinking [or] to begin exercising?"

Another predictor of success is the patient's self-efficacy regarding change. Self-efficacy is typically assessed relative to a specific task or situation. Asking questions such as "How confident do you feel that you can turn down a cigarette if a coworker offers one to you?" will provide a good estimate. Depending upon the patient's responsiveness, it may be helpful to discuss strategies for these situations and even to role-play these challenges to encourage the patient to practice successful responses.

Arrange

After discussing concrete strategies for change (Assist), close follow-up should be arranged. The scheduling of follow-up contact may differ depending on the problem type and the patient's apparent ability to enact the recommended plan. For example, nicotine withdrawal during smoking cessation includes unpleasant physical and emotional reactions. While the worst of these experiences usually lasts 24–72 hours after the last cigarette, withdrawal symptoms may be present, to some degree, for 2–3 weeks before they abate. With smoking cessation, it is helpful to see the patient or speak by phone during the first week and to see them a second time during the first month (Fiore et al., 2000). During the second and third months, periodic supportive contact with a psychologist by phone or trained office staff increases the likelihood of successful cessation.

Application of the Five "A"s

Panic Disorder

While the five "A"s are generally employed for health risk behaviors and control of chronic illness, Hunter et al. (2009) have used this approach to address panic disorder. In the initial phase, targeted questions are asked such as

> Have you ever had an episode when you suddenly felt your heart racing, had difficulty breathing, started feeling shaky or dizzy, and you were worried that you might die, suffocate, or something bad would happen? (Hunter et al., 2009).

In the advice phase, the possibility of selective serotonin reuptake inhibitors (SSRIs), education about panic disorder, as well as cognitive-behavioral self-control techniques, are presented to the patient. Cognitive-behavioral techniques appear to be optimally helpful for longer-term relief of panic symptoms. A highlight of the agreement phase is determining whether the patient would be able and willing to tolerate some of the physiological symptoms for a period of time until they are under better control through cognitive-behavioral methods. For example, relaxation techniques are often helpful but require practice and may not eliminate symptoms.

Education also assists patients in managing their panic attacks. Specifically the psychologist may provide written information indicating that the symptoms are not due to a more serious medical condition – an ongoing concern of patients with panic attacks (Hunter et al., 2009). At that point, cognitive interventions including acceptance and commitment therapy (see Chapter 8) may be employed. Additionally gradual exposure to environments associated with attacks as well as interoceptive exposure is recommended. Interoceptive exposure involves deliberately provoking some of the physical symptoms of panic, such as increased heart rate by running up multiple flights of stairs or producing shortness of breath through hyperventilation. The goal is for the patient to be able to tolerate these physical sensations as well as underscoring that these experiences are not life threatening. Additionally, because it involves bringing symptoms on through the patient's efforts, interoceptive exposure emphasizes that the patient does have some degree of voluntary control over these unpleasant physical sensations. This aspect is particularly important since panic symptoms often seem to come "out of the blue" and are experienced as uncontrollable. Finally, the arrange phase may not be necessary since the combination of SSRIs and cognitive-behavioral techniques, particularly interoceptive exposure, will make symptoms at least manageable for the majority of patients. However, among patients with continued and more intractable episodes of panic, referral to a specialty mental health provider should be considered. In keeping with a stepped care approach, for the small minority of patients who do not respond to first-line therapy, combination pharmacotherapy of two psychotropic medications and/or more extended cognitive-behavioral treatment, with an exposure component, from a therapist specializing in anxiety disorders, may be necessary.

Health Promotion
The benefits of physical activity appear to be significant in reducing cardiovascular risk factors including metabolism, blood pressure, insulin utilization as well as improved efficiency of skeletal muscle blood flow. Research has suggested that even in the absence of significant weight loss, patients predisposed to developing type II diabetes can improve cardiovascular functioning and reduce their risk regardless of whether exercise is associated with significant weight loss. Other data indicate that physical activity improves psychological well-being and that those engaged in regular exercise have fewer sick days (Peterson, 2007). Primary care research has found that patients receiving only 3–5 minutes of physical activity counseling improved their activity level (specifically increased their number of minutes per week of walking) relative to those who received typical care. Other studies have found that patients who were briefly counseled about exercise, including both advice and assistance (two of the "A"s), had higher levels of cardiovascular fitness than those receiving advice alone.

Ask (Assess)
When asked directly, patients tend to be fairly straightforward in reporting their level of physical activity. The only common ambiguity is that patients often indicate that they believe that they get adequate physical activity walking to their office from the parking lot or ambling through a store. Prior to initiating an exercise program, patients should be screened the possibility of a coronary event. This is particularly true for patients with a history of heart disease or diabetes. A useful screening tool is the Physical Activity

Readiness Questionnaire (Canadian Society for Exercise Physiology, 1994). This questionnaire asks the patients if they had ever been told by a physician that they have heart problems, whether they are currently having pains in their heart and chest, have a history of high blood pressure, are over age 60 and not used to vigorous exercise, or have had recent episodes of dizziness. If the patient does endorse one of these items, it is recommended that they receive a more thorough medical evaluation before initiating exercise. The primary care psychologist should be aware that it is advisable for patients who have not exercised on a regular basis or those with a history of cardiovascular disease to be medically cleared prior to initiating regular physical activity. Clearance may include cardiac stress testing prior to regular exercise (Peterson, 2007).

Advise

In advising about physical activity level, there are three key parameters: frequency, intensity, and duration. Frequency is reflected in the number of days a week that the patient will be active; duration is the amount of time spent in activity per session, and intensity is the level of effort (Peterson, 2007). Moderate intensity of activity includes activities such as brisk walking at a speed of 3–4 mph, bicycling, and vacuuming or mowing the lawn. For patients who have been inactive, it is suggested that they begin with approximately 10 minutes per day and add 10-minute increments every 1–2 weeks with the goal of 30 minutes of activity daily. Again it is often helpful to provide the patient with an individualized handout addressing the important aspects of exercise initiation.

Agree

In order to document physical activity, it is recommended that patients be encouraged to maintain a physical activity log which they may also bring to follow-up visits. The fitness plan should be realistically matched to the patient's lifestyle. For example, patients who enjoy watching television might be more likely to work out regularly if they put a stationary bike in front of the television.

Assist

In terms of assistance, there is considerable evidence that the presence of social support – such as a spouse or friend who will walk regularly with the patient – is particularly helpful in carrying out a physical activity program. The other key component of this phase is to ask the patient if there are any particular obstacles that may prevent them from carrying out their exercise plan. It is also helpful to talk with patients about how they will handle obstacles such as when they feel too fatigued to exercise or are distracted by other activities. Importantly, they should have a plan for getting back into their exercise routine should they fall away for several days to a week.

Arrange

Arranging should include follow-up contact that includes attention to the patient's exercise goal. This support can be by telephone but should include some in person visits to which the patient brings their completed exercise logs. In reviewing the log, attention should be devoted to any periods in which the patient was inactive for multiple days. These difficulties can become a focus of problem solving regarding barriers (Peterson, 2007).

Research on the Five "A"s

Counseling patients on the five "A"s, as described in the beginning of the chapter, typically requires less than 15 minutes. Research with pregnant smokers found that use of the five "A"s was associated with greater cessation rates than the physician's recommendation, alone. In most research demonstrating the effectiveness of the five "As," providers have been primary care physicians. Among a group of obstetricians, the prenatal providers rated their own skills as generally good in counseling with the five "A"s around tobacco use during pregnancy. The physicians reported being less comfortable, but generally able, to use the five "A"s in evaluating drug and alcohol use. They reported less confidence and greater discomfort in implementing the technique to address possible domestic violence (Herzig et al., 2006).

This exception is noteworthy since domestic violence is a risk factor that increases during pregnancy. Surveys suggest that female patients are not disturbed by questions about violence if raised with concern and compassion. Providers expressed some dissonance regarding alcohol use during pregnancy. While they felt compelled to explain the current American College of Obstetricians and Gynecologists recommendations that pregnant women abstain from alcohol completely during pregnancy, several reported that they, personally, were not convinced that low-level drinking had adverse fetal effects (Herzig et al., 2006).

FRAMES

FRAMES is an acronym (**F**eedback, **R**esponsibility, **A**dvice, **M**enu of strategies, **E**mpathy, **S**elf-efficacy) that was originally developed as an efficient protocol for primary care physicians to address excessive alcohol use in their patients (NIAAA, 1999). It shares some similarities with the five "A"s as well as with the stages of change and motivational interviewing discussed in the next two chapters. However, FRAMES was developed for physicians rather than psychologists, and assumes that patients with substance abuse and noncompliance will present with physical or laboratory findings related to substance use.

Feedback

The encounter begins by providing the patient with concrete feedback. This is typically in the form of laboratory results such as abnormal liver function tests or elevated blood pressure (associated with alcohol abuse), chronic respiratory symptoms (associated with smoking), or measures of blood sugar such as hemoglobin A-1 C (used to assess diabetic adherence over a 3-month period). Summary scores on screening measures such as the CAGE or the Fagerstrom Index (described in Chapter 4) may also be used. However, there is a preference for "hard data" such as physiological abnormalities.

The provider then makes a very specific link between the patient's risk behavior and their physical health status. If the patient has a high hemoglobin A-1 C value indicative of poor diabetic control, the provider will discuss the meaning of that indicator and also describe long-range effects of poor diabetic control such as retinopathy and peripheral neuropathy. If alcohol abuse is the issue, the provider may say: "One thing we do know is that patients who drink more than three drinks a day have a much higher rate of health problems including hypertension and liver disease."

Responsibility

Responsibility for change resides with the patient. The health care provider conveys this attitude in multiple ways. For example, when presenting feedback, the provider does not automatically assume that the patient wants to make the changes necessary to improve their health status. However, in contrast to more complex models of counseling such as motivational interviewing, the patient's responsibility is explicitly stated. Provider statements such as "You have the ultimate control over your drinking or smoking ..." or "How long do you think you'll continue smoking?" (Searight, 2007) or "Change is up to you." emphasize patients' responsibility. A somewhat less confrontational tone may be used by borrowing some of the verbal strategies from motivational interviewing. Statements such as "What are your thoughts about getting your blood sugar under better control?" and "Is this a concern for you?" convey that it is the patient's choice about whether to address the health concern. If the patient appears uncomfortable, they should be asked directly about this: "Are you comfortable with this discussion, do you want to continue?" If the patient says they do not want to continue the discussion, the clinician should respond by asking them if it would be okay to raise the issue at their next visit.

Advice to Change

In the FRAMES protocol, the physician provides direct advice. "For your health, I strongly recommend that you take your blood pressure medication every day as we discussed." or "To avoid later complications of diabetes" I strongly recommend that you stay on an appropriate diabetic diet and take your blood sugar readings every day according to the schedule that we have discussed. For many psychologists, this approach may seem somewhat heavy-handed. However, it should be remembered that patients are typically in a state of distress and anxiety when seeing the physician. The physician can capitalize on their authority at these times and have maximal influence over patient behavior.

Menu of Strategies

In following the protocol sequentially, it is noteworthy that the patient's responsibility is stressed immediately before the provider's directive and then again immediately afterward.

The patient's responsibility is further underscored by providing them with as many concrete strategies for change as is feasible. Patients with obesity may be advised about the availability of weight loss medications, calorie counting diet programs such as Weight Watchers, and/or regular aerobic exercise. Similarly for smoking cessation, the patient can be provided with information about pharmacotherapy including nicotine replacement as well as stimulus control approaches and support groups. The patient is encouraged to select the options which best fit with their lifestyle (Searight, 2007).

Empathy

There is a growing body of research on physician communication indicating that patients are more likely to follow advice when the physician conveys empathy. The importance of empathy is well known to psychologists and is part of any successful approach to psychotherapy or counseling. Importantly, for patients who are engaging in behavior such as drinking or smoking, it is helpful to ask about the needs that are being met through these activities. Again this should be done in an inquisitive, nonjudgmental manner. (What do you like about drinking – is there anything that you could put it in place of the three beers after work?) The provider also seems more genuine and credible if they can convey some appreciation of how difficult these lifestyle changes are to make. (Quitting smoking after all these years will be really hard. It sounds like you appreciate how tough those first few days without a cigarette can be (Searight, 2007, 2009).)

Self-efficacy

Finally, as in the five "A"s, it is important to affirm the patient's strengths. Verbally indicating that the provider respects the patient's desire and motivation to change, by itself, will be experienced as supportive. Another useful strategy is to ask the patient what they would see as a reasonable short-term goal. This built-in accountability also conveys the provider's optimism that the patient will can be successful (NIAAA, 1999). Importantly, however, the patient should take the lead in setting this goal since that will promote personal ownership as well as make it more likely that the patient will experience confidence in achieving it.

Follow-up is also important. Patients' successes should be emphasized. For example, even if the patient lapses after 2 months of being cigarette free, the clinician can point out that the patient has been successful in getting through the most difficult time period, which is typically the 2 weeks immediately following cessation in which nicotine withdrawal is most pronounced. The patient should, as with the five "A"s, be encouraged to keep a log of smoking, alcohol, diet, or exercise. If a review of these patient-completed records indicates that the patient is not following through with the plan, the provider should cycle back to the "M" (menu) and discuss alternatives that might work better now that the patient has additional knowledge of the challenges involved in changing.

Evidence for FRAMES

While the FRAMES method, per se, has not been widely evaluated, the basic components of FRAMES – and in particular, brief intervention – do have a reasonable evidence basis. For example, an empathetic counseling style was found to be more effective in reducing drinking. Patients whose counselors employed an empathetic style were more likely to reduce their alcohol consumption compared with counselors using a more confrontational approach (77% vs. 55%) (Miller & Rollnick, 2004). This type of intervention has also been used in emergency departments with patients who have alcohol-related injuries. Evidence, to date suggests that brief intervention, similar to FRAMES, is associated with reduced alcohol consumption as well as fewer adverse alcohol-related consequences (D'Onofrio & Degutis, 2004). Physician counseling coupled with nicotine replacement therapy was found to be associated with greater smoking abstinence at both 6 and 12 months. The elements of the counseling model were similar to FRAMES in that it was patient centered, addressed current concerns as well as past experiences with smoking and cessation, developed a concrete plan for change, and provided appropriate follow-up (Ockene et al., 1994).

While perhaps counterintuitive to many psychologists, research on brief interventions for alcohol abuse has found that, at least in primary care settings, there appear to be minimal differences between outcomes for brief and longer-term treatments for alcohol abuse and problem drinking (Moyer, Finney, Swearingen, & Vergun, 2002).

Conclusion

The interventions described in this chapter may seem almost minuscule to many psychologists. However, when applied to specific health risk factors – most notably alcohol abuse – they do appear to be effective in reducing alcohol consumption as well as in reducing alcohol-related health problems. While both of these models – the five "A"s and FRAMES – can be adapted to longer-term interventions such as focused cognitive-behavioral treatment of panic disorder, brief problem-focused counseling is acceptable to a wide array of patients. Additionally, these approaches have demonstrated effectiveness for reducing, but not eliminating, health risk behavior in the primary care sector.

Chapter 6

Assessing and Addressing Patient Motivation With the Stages of Change

The Rise of Nonadherence as a Pervasive Health Problem

Since the early 20th century there has been a major change in causes of morbidity and mortality from acute infectious diseases such as tuberculosis to chronic illness such as cardiovascular disease. As Cassell (1997) notes, while infectious disease is still present, it no longer occupies a central position in Western medicine. As a result, primary health care, rather than being disease oriented, is increasingly focused on disability. Another key distinction is that while acute illnesses are treated in the clinic by health care professionals, chronic illnesses are principally treated by patients, themselves. While "compliance" is still often used to describe the phenomenon of following health care recommendations, "adherence" is becoming the preferred term since it suggests a collaborative partnership between physician and patient. Maintaining appointments, taking medication on a regular basis, reducing exposure to harmful influences such as cigarette smoke, excess alcohol, and high-fat food as well as health-promoting activities such as exercise and diet, all fall under the patient's, rather than the provider's control.

With this rise in chronic illness as the principal source of morbidity and mortality in the United States, the focus in medicine is now on preventing illness as well as reducing the development of further symptoms in those already affected. A central issue is that despite the fact that health risks, medications, and lifestyle prescriptions are well known to the general public, the rate of chronic illness and accompanying complications continues to rise. A central dilemma is that knowledge of health-promoting activity does not translate into day-to-day action. For example, among patients with diabetes, it was found that 80% were administering their insulin incorrectly while nearly 60% were not taking the correct dose and over three-quarters were taking blood glucose readings incorrectly with a similar percentage not following prescribed dietary guidelines (D'Eramo-Melkus & Demas, 1989; Searight, 1999).

This dilemma has led to a central problem in health communication: How do clinicians motivate people to comply with recommendations and established public health guidelines? Both models of counseling discussed in this and in the following chapter address the issue of patient motivation. These approaches assume that patients must undergo cognitive changes in their evaluation of health risks and the extent to which they view these risks as personally applicable. Once changes in belief systems occur, the patient's health behavior will follow.

The Transtheoretical Model and the Stages of Change

Overview

The Transtheoretical Model (TM) assumes that health behavior change occurs in stages reflecting various levels of patient motivation and perceived self-efficacy. These stages are Precontemplation, Contemplation, Preparation, Action, and Maintenance. Progressing through the stages depends upon the cognitive balance between the "pros" and "cons" of change. Direct advice or education alone is assumed to be ineffective until the patient has moved to a later stage in which they are ready to act. The clinician attempts to match their communication to the patient's stage. Through targeted questions, the patient's reasons for change come to outweigh the barriers to the point where they are ready to take action. TM, originally developed for smoking cessation, has been adapted to a range of other problems including exercise initiation, reduction in excess dietary fat, weight loss, alcohol cessation, marijuana use, adherence with a treatment plan, safe sex, and sunscreen use (Prochaska et al., 1994). Each of these stages will be discussed below.

Precontemplation

The formal definition of Precontemplation is a state in which the patient has no plans to change the target health behavior within the next 6 months (Prochaska, Redding, & Evers, 2008). In this stage, clinician counseling should focus upon increasing the patient's motivation for change (Katz, 2001). Typically, the precontemplative patient has given little or no thought to changing. The absence of interest may stem from a perception that the behavior is not harmful and/or is not something that can be changed. It is also possible that patients may have an awareness that habits such as smoking are harmful but maintain this recognition at an unconscious level. Once people engaging in health risk behavior are aware of its harm, they may selectively ignore information or cognitively move themselves out of the at-risk category. ("other people become dependent on alcohol to make it through the day; I don't have that problem – I could quit anytime I want to.")

For the clinician, the challenge in communicating with a patient at this stage is to increase their awareness of the harm associated with their habit but without eliciting too much anxiety. Moderate anxiety is probably optimal – there has to be enough of a threat to get the patient's attention and arouse some discomfort. However, arousing too much anxiety will result in the patient shutting down and being less likely to follow up with the provider. On the other hand, colluding with the patient's silence about their behavior is similarly harmful. If a health care professional does not remark on their continued smoking, the patient experiences support in their view that their habit is nothing to worry about.

Effective communication with precontemplators centers around acknowledging the risky behavior and letting the patient know that when they are ready to address it, you are available. In patients seen over the course of multiple months to several years, the issue should be raised at subsequent health care visits but in the spirit of "are you ready, yet?" When the patient indicates that they are still not interested in changing, the provider does not press the issue but still communicates that it is important – "When smoking is something you want to discuss further, please let me know and if its ok, I will check in with you about it the next time we meet." Some physicians "flag" patients' charts with special stickers to remind them to ask about smoking at each visit.

Some patients may be unaware that their behavior is harmful. An example is smoking cigarettes or marijuana or daily alcohol use among pregnant women. Many women believe that low levels of substance use do not pose any harm to the developing fetus. In these circumstances, because the urgency is greater, the clinician should provide factual information about the risks of continuing substance use during pregnancy (e.g., lower birth weight infants among pregnant smokers) and follow up with exploratory questions such as "What do you like about smoking?"; "How long do you think you will keep smoking?"; and "What would tell you that it might be time to stop?" (Searight, 2007, 2009). These questions are also useful for follow-up visits for all patients in this stage.

Precontemplative patients who have made previous quit attempts should be encouraged to describe previous efforts, with particular attention to the methods used, environmental obstacles, and the duration of success. In counseling these patients, it will be necessary to look for indicators that something has changed so that the next attempt will be more successful. The change may be a lesson learned from the relapse. However the patient may have emerged from their relapse with a pessimistic view of their own ability to be successful. Counseling should focus upon understanding any environmental obstacles that occurred during the previous attempt as well as listening for ways in which the patient's perspective on the problem can change so that they feel a greater sense of self-efficacy (Katz, 2001).

Contemplation

In this stage, the patient is considering changing their behavior within the next 6 months. The provider should keep in mind the key word "considering" – this is not yet a final decision with an accompanying plan. As will be discussed further in the next chapter, ambivalence characterizes nearly all attempts at significant health behavior change. In this stage, the desire for change and resistance to change have nearly equal influence (Katz, 2001). Counseling can increase the motivation for change or decrease the barriers and/ or perceived disadvantages of change. Some useful questions are "What advantages do you see in changing?"; "What disadvantages do you see in changing?"; What would be the hardest part of changing?"; "Do you see any other advantages to changing?"; and "What could get in the way of changing?" (Searight, 2007, 2009).

Preparation

In Preparation, the patient has made a decision to change in the next 30 days. They are developing a plan that includes concrete, specific activities. Evidence of Preparation might include visiting several commercial gyms for an exercise program, signing up for a weight reduction program, or obtaining information on diabetic or low-fat diets. With smoking cessation, patients in this stage typically have chosen a quit date. In this stage, the focus of counseling should be on potential obstacles. In addition, beginning discussion of possible high-risk situations which could provoke lapses is also helpful. For patients who have selected a specific quit date, it is helpful to ask them how they chose that particular day. For example, if the smoker has targeted the day that a smoking ban in the workplace will go into effect, it would be beneficial to encourage the patient to begin taking one fewer smoke break per day or several fewer smoke breaks per week during the upcoming month. In addition, if the patient cannot describe an alternative plan for breaks at work, they should be encouraged to develop one. As a general rule, patients should be reminded that it is difficult to simply stop a behavior without putting something else in its place. If not already discussed, specific, implementable alternatives should be developed. Many patients do not have well thought out plans for smoking cessation or dieting but will simply say "I'm going to use my 'will power'." While affirming the patient's motivation, the clinician should explore ways in which their environment may support or hinder the change process. One useful question in this stage is "Do you foresee any situations where you might be tempted to start overeating/smoking/drinking?"

Action

In this stage, patients are actively changing. Contact with the patient during this stage, in which the change has been in place for under 6 months (Prochaska et al., 2008), is particularly important for both general support and to target any unanticipated difficulties that have arisen. Useful questions for the Action phase include "How is the plan working?"; "Has anything come up that you didn't expect?" Asking about lapses or temptations to lapse will provide useful information about unforeseen challenges. This dynamic will be discussed further below. Lapses should be viewed as normal and as part of the change process. For patients who did briefly lapse, their coping skills can be affirmed by asking "How did you get back on track?" (Searight, 2007, 2009). Additionally, lapses typically provide information about high-risk situations that were not anticipated. The patient should be asked what they learned from the experience.

Maintenance

Maintenance is the 6-month period immediately following Action in which the patient successfully continues their behavior change. Supportive statements highlighting the patient's coping skills are important. Counseling should emphasize that success has been due to the patient's efforts rather than circumstances, the effects of medication, or luck. Paying particular attention to the patient's control validates their self-efficacy and increases the likelihood that they will use active problem-solving strategies when confronted with a challenge to their new lifestyle. The keys to successful Maintenance are well-developed relapse prevention strategies.

The following sections examine in more detail the actual processes involved in moving from one stage to the next. The more recent addition of a specific relapse prevention approach (Marlatt & Donovan, 2005) to the stages model is consistent with research indicating that success is not a discontinuous, "all or nothing" phenomenon.

The Process of Moving Through the Stages

Evidence suggests that movement from Preparation to Action depends upon the balance between the patient's perceived advantages (pros) and barriers (cons) to change. Patients may be in the Precontemplation stage for one of three reasons. They may (1) fail to recognize that their behavior is a problem (some of these patients may respond to a more directive, educational approach such as the five "A"s or FRAMES); (2) not perceive the risk to be personally applicable (I drank during my other two pregnancies. The kids are fine.) even though objectively recognizing that the behavior is considered unhealthy; and (3) be undecided and "stuck" with an unprioritized set of pros and cons.

Moving to Contemplation requires an increase in the number of "pros" for change. Research suggests that this shift may be problem dependent. For sunscreen use, mammography, and lower-fat diets, the pros of changing did not outweigh the cons of remaining the same until the Action stage (Prochaska et al., 1994). In moving from Precontemplation to Contemplation, communication should focus on the advantages (pros) of change. Once the patient accepts these "pros," the clinician's targeted questions shift to reducing the perceived disadvantages of change.

Once the barriers to change are reduced, patients are able to prepare for Action. As compared with the earlier stages, during Preparation, patients are more likely to be open to advice and concrete assistance. This may include pharmacotherapy for smoking cessation or a referral to a nutritionist for weight loss. During Action and Maintenance, patients may briefly lapse or experience a more enduring relapse. Instead of communicating disappointment, psychologists should normalize these episodes as part of the change process. For example, the average cigarette smoker has approximately six quit episodes before lifetime cessation.

Kaizen

During either the Contemplation or the Preparation stages, patients often benefit from initiating action on a very reduced scale. Kaizen, a technique originally associated with management, encourages taking very small steps toward personal goals rather than viewing change as requiring a massive restructuring of one's lifestyle (Maurer, 2004). Kaizen came from the need to rapidly improve production in US industries during the Second World War. Since there was no time for large-scale changes in production, machinery, processes, or management, a policy of continuous improvement was recommended. Given the circumstances, being alert to the number of very small ways that efficiency could be enhanced was seen as the only realistic approach. Kaizen was introduced by the US to postwar Japan and has been cited as a key force in the dramatic rise in Japan as a world economic force (Maurer, 2004).

At an individual level, Kaizen encourages beginning the process of behavior change with small, seemingly trivial, acts that are consistent with the desired goal. Recognizing the evidence that plans for self-improvement involving large-scale lifestyle changes are either not initiated or maintained, this approach begins with minimal efforts. For someone who has been completely sedentary for years, a directive to walk briskly for 30 minutes/day four times per week will seem like a huge challenge which will be intimidating to start and is unlikely to be maintained.

Instead, suggesting that the patient walk 5 minutes per day – even less – in place while watching television is much more likely to be successful (Maurer, 2004). Gradually, the patient's walking time can be increased by 1–2 minutes per week. Since they are able to achieve initial goals and because the next level is experienced as a minimal increase, patients can readily comply. If the patient experiences their eating as "out of control," ask them to throw away the first bite of their snack. These small successes lead to enhanced self-efficacy which becomes a force for further change (Maurer, 2004).

Maurer (2004) describes some useful questions that can provoke productive planning. For patients who are depressed, feeling overwhelmed, or struggling with chronic illness "If you were guaranteed not to fail, what would [you] be doing differently?" (p. 63). For those interested in, but anxious about, making a lifestyle change, "What is one small step [you] could make toward reaching [your] goal?" (Maurer, p. 64). Once the change process has begun – even on a miniscule level – the consideration of pros and cons that moves patients through the stages also becomes less overwhelming.

Cognitive and Emotional Factors in the Stages of Change

During the Precontemplation and Contemplation stages, patients are more likely to respond to a cognitive approach such as a discussion of the benefits of habit change possibly supported by written information. In Preparation, the focus will turn to the disadvantages of changing. While these might include intrapersonal experiences (e.g., increased anxiety if the patient no longer drinks in the evening), they are also likely to include social pressures. ("The guys at work will think I'm being stuck up if I don't go on smoke break with them.") Both aversive mood states and interpersonal dynamics are powerful forces. The provider and patient should develop a concrete and realistic plan for addressing these concerns given the patient's life circumstances. For example, developing alternative strategies for managing tension after work without drinking might include taking a walk or engaging in a hobby such as woodworking or gardening. For the social pressures associated with smoking, the provider and patient can role-play ways that the patient can communicate a desire to stay socially engaged with coworkers while avoiding environmental cues for cigarettes. The Action stage should target the behavioral skills and day-to-day challenges the patient encounters (Searight, 2007). In these patient discussions, the psychologist should be careful to avoid moving through the stages too quickly and miss cues that the patient is still in an earlier stage. This mismatched communication is likely to leave the patient feeling misunderstood which may be reflected in failure to follow up.

Maintenance, Lapse, and Relapse

There has been increased recognition that Maintenance is a much more dynamic process than originally described. In the early 1970s, Marlatt (Marlatt & Witkiewitz, 2005) examined factors associated with initiating drinking among patients during the first 90 days after inpatient substance abuse treatment. Beliefs about successful coping were, as would be expected, predictive of whether patients would reinitiate drinking. However, initial slips or lapses are highly probable in most attempts at behavior change.

A key factor is determining when these lapses become a more enduring relapse. Some patients are able to lapse and get themselves back on track fairly quickly while for others, the lapse begins a fairly rapid return to previous high-risk behavior. One key determinant may be "the abstinence violation effect," a sense of self-blame and failure and perceived loss of control (Marlatt & Donovan, 2005). This effect can be interpreted catastrophically "It just proves that I can't quit smoking – no matter what I do. I might just as well stop trying to quit and accept that I'll be a two pack a day smoker the rest of my life." The interpretation of these episodes of absence of control and/or diminished coping skills is the key factor in determining whether someone will "get back on the wagon" or will go into a downward spiral of substance use. The experience of craving – the intense desire for the banned substance or activity – appears to interact with the availability of the forbidden substance and, in the face of poor coping skills, contributes to the deterioration of self-control. Research does suggest that patients can clearly label high- and low-risk situations (Witkiewitz & Marlatt, 2004). While self-regulation is important, abstinence is also influenced by environmental factors. When self-regulation resources are repeatedly challenged by environmental cues (e.g., for a smoker, presence of cigarettes, lighters, and a spouse who smokes) there is an experience of self-regulation fatigue.

These findings lead to important directions for brief intervention. First, it is important to encourage the patient to predict possible lapse situations for the future and help develop a strategy that can be implemented when craving begins. Cravings are time limited – often the most intense desire for cigarettes, alcohol, or high-fat food – last 10 minutes or less. However, for the patient attempting self-control, these relatively brief time frames are experienced as interminable. Importantly, they are analogous to putting one's hand on a hot stove; the intensity of these cravings is so powerful that the patient feels that they must act immediately in response (Marlatt & Witkiewitz, 2005). The most helpful skills at these times are to physically remove oneself from the stimuli-inducing craving and/or using cognitive skills to transform the stimuli into something far less appetitive. For example, asking the patient to imagine picking up a cigarette butt out of a pool of vomit on the sidewalk to smoke it is likely to produce initial revulsion.

However over time, even in the presence of strong self-regulation skills, continued environmental stimulation is likely to produce restraint fatigue. From a practical perspective, patients should be encouraged to have an advance plan to eventually remove themselves from high-risk situations when they arise.

Importantly, lapses are to be expected. Research as well as narrative accounts of success in smoking cessation, sobriety, or diet, all include episodes of "falling off the wagon." This raises a dilemma in counseling patients. Since lapses are to be expected, should they be predicted for the patient or does this prediction, in and of itself, become a self-fulfilling prophecy? Once the patient has lapsed or relapsed, it is important that they consider the situation and use it as a learning experience. For example, a problem drinker, who consumed several beers in response to social pressure or began drinking heavily before stopping the next day, should address several issues. First, helping them identify the triggers (I'm sure I can just drink one beer without going back to heavy drinking) as well as the process by which they became abstinent again can consolidate coping skills. Being able to articulate these threats, the accompanying thought processes, and similarly being able to describe successful coping to get "back on the wagon," will help the patient the next time these challenges arise. Particularly in working with patients who have succeeded in overcoming a lapse, the psychologist may be reluctant to examine the episode in much detail for fear of emphasizing the patient's failure and diminishing self-efficacy. However, if approached in the right spirit ("This sounds like a situation that you didn't expect. You know, its too bad that we can't predict every challenge that you will come up against. However, we can learn from them."), the patient will experience support and confidence in their ability to address future threats.

When patients were able to circumscribe the lapse and prevent themselves from returning to the habit, asking them about the strategies they used to regain successful coping will also help concretize these skills so that they can be used in the future. In addition, highlighting this eventual victory will offset temporarily, diminished self-efficacy.

When patients are having more struggles with lapses, several counseling techniques are useful. First, accepting that they may give in to temptation, but encouraging them to give in less (stop at 10 cookies instead of 20, 10 cigarettes per day instead of the whole pack). The ability to keep from returning to previous levels demonstrates some level of self-control and reduces the catastrophic reaction to abstinence violation. Second, if lapses are not diminishing in frequency, another strategy is to ask the patient to wait 5–10 minutes before giving in. This approach communicates several messages – the craving is not as powerful as believed since they can wait before acting on it, some remnant of self-control remains, and distraction for brief periods of time can be effective. Moreover, the patient may be able to distract themselves so successfully that they make it through the most intense period of craving without giving in and become absorbed in the distracting activity (a television show, a book, conversation with a friend).

Recently, a systematic approach to responding to potential high-risk situations has been supported. Armitage (2008) worked with smokers and developed a volitional help sheet, a set of intentions to be employed in high-risk situations. The help sheet lists 20 high-risk situations for reinitiating smoking (e.g., "If I am tempted to smoke in a bar or pub having a drink...."; "If I am tempted to smoke when I feel I need a lift...."; "If I am tempted to smoke with my partner or close friend who is smoking...") (Armitage, 2008, p. 566). In addition, it lists out 20 potential solutions (e.g., "Then I will do something else instead of smoking;" "Then I will stop to think that smoking is polluting the environment"). In using the sheet, smokers make a link between specific situations that they confront and solutions that they believe would be effective in addressing these challenges. Some examples: If "I am tempted to smoke over coffee while talking and relaxing".... then "I will seek out someone who listens when I need to talk about my smoking." If "I'm tempted to smoke when I first get up in the morning" then "I will tell myself if I try hard enough I can keep from smoking." If "I'm tempted to smoke when I'm extremely anxious and stressed" then "I will remember that my need for cigarettes makes me feel disappointed in myself." (Armitage, 2008, p. 566). It was found that this approach was more effective in maintaining cessation compared with simply noting high-risk situations and adaptive responses without specifically linking them (Armitage, 2008). This effect is likely attributable to the fact that it gives the patient a set of personally specific strategies that are automatically available in situations where lapse is likely.

Stages of Change and Chronic Illness

With the complicated behavioral regimen often required for managing chronic illness such as asthma, hypertension, and type II diabetes, patients often have varying levels of mastery for specific aspects of self-management. For example, with the asthmatic child, the use of a maintenance inhaler is important and prevents inappropriate and early use of a rescue inhaler when symptoms occur. Other issues include minimizing contact with potential irritants such as cigarette smoke, pet dander, and dust. With patients managing type II diabetes, there are several key behaviors including maintaining an appropriate diet, engaging in regular physical activity, taking medication regularly and in some cases, taking blood sugar readings. Those who have attempted to apply the stages of change model to chronic illness suggest that patients may be in various stages with respect to some of the specific behaviors. For example, an individual may be in Contemplation regarding physical activity, Maintenance with respect to blood glucose testing, and Contemplation about a specific diet.

Research on the Stages of Change

While the concept of patients being at varying levels of readiness to change does appear to have fairly solid empirical support, interventions based upon this model have yielded less consistent findings. In large samples of smokers, 40% were in Precontemplation, 40% in Contemplation, and 20% in Preparation (Velcier et al., 1995). Prochaska et al. (1994)

conducted a large-scale review and found that the stage model could explain 12 different problem behaviors ranging from cocaine use to cigarette smoking to adolescent delinquency, mammography, condom use, weight control, and high-fat diets. The balance between pros and cons generally followed the predictions of the model. For example, for all of the behaviors, the cons of changing outweighed the pros during the Precontemplation stage while in the Action stage, the pros predominated for nearly all behaviors with cocaine use being the only exception. Of interest, the shift between pros and cons occurred during Precontemplation for 7 of the 12 behaviors. This shift occurred during the Action stage for sunscreen use, high-fat diets, mammography, and delinquency. For exercise initiation, this shift occurred during the Preparation stage. However on the whole, the model accounted for behavior change or lack thereof for a broad cross-section of diverse health behaviors.

For some behaviors, there is evidence that relapse and previous quit attempts – particularly if recent – increase motivation to move from Contemplation into Preparation. For example among smokers, a recent quit attempt leading to relapse seemed to be associated with greater movement through the Contemplation and onto the Preparation stage. However, there also appeared to be a group of "chronic contemplators" who had difficulty moving to the next step (DiClemente et al., 1991).

The relationship between lapse and relapse, as described above, also has evidence-based support. Among women who were in a 14-week exercise program, over 60% lapsed at some point. Among that group, 41% had a 3-week consecutive relapse episode. Of note, those who reported better coping skills were more likely to return to exercise after the lapse compared with those who relapsed (Simkin & Gross, 1994). For practitioners, this pattern suggests that time spent discussing threats to maintenance as well as life circumstances that could lead to a lapse, and then discussing alternative coping responses, can be valuable. For substance use, high-risk situations for relapse typically include both intrapersonal and interpersonal factors. Emotional states such as depression and anxiety were described as much more predictive of relapse than cravings. Among a group of dieters, positive emotional states were more predictive of relapse than cravings (Collins, 2005).

Support for tailored communication in which communication to the patient is matched to their current stage is less consistent. For example, in a review of research on stage-based dietary intervention for diabetes, findings were mixed. In comparing patients who had received stage-based feedback with those receiving typical care, there were differences in favor of the stage group in terms of total fat intake, monosaturated fat intake, and systolic blood pressure. However, there were no differences on a wide variety of other indices including weight, diastolic blood pressure, unsaturated fat intake, overall blood pressure, waist-to-hip ratio, as well as amount of weight regained after the initial loss (Salmela, Poskiparta, Kasila, Vahasarja, & Vanhala, 2008).

However, a recent population-based study did find support for stage-based intervention for a range of health-related behaviors (Johnson et al., 2007). In a large group of overweight or obese adults, interventions targeted multiple behaviors related to weight management. Stage-based counseling was provided through individualized, tailored, computer-generated reports matching recommendations for activity to the patient's current stage. Behaviors of interest included healthy eating, exercise, and managing emotional distress – all of which demonstrated greater improvement in the stages intervention. While these behaviors changed by 6 months, significant weight loss was not evident until approximately 24 months. Weight loss is likely the result of multiple behavior changes and as noted above, patients may be in various stages with respect to each. The stage-based feedback was also successful in moving patients from earlier stages to Action and Maintenance. The authors point out that at a population level, the average number of changes per person was significantly greater than that reported for previous studies focusing on a single health behavior. While the average number of changes per person in a stage-based smoking cessation study was one per five participants, in this study the average number of behaviors changed per person was three per four individuals. At a population level, addressing multiple behaviors, over time, is likely to have greater impact than focusing on one behavior, alone, to reduce health risk (Johnson et al., 2007).

Conclusion

Historically, the TM was important because it described change as a series of processes rather than an all-or-nothing event. With the addition of the decisional balance dimensions of the pros and cons of changing, the model described a systematic and logical approach to moving from Precontemplation to Action and onto permanent change. Like all stage theories, there is a degree of artificiality in assuming that people abruptly and linearly move discontinuously toward health. More recent formulations suggest that people may cycle through the stages multiple times, and if they have gone through the sequence once, may start again at a later point in the chain when they address a habit that has returned. The later addition of lapse and relapse theory captures how change actually occurs – through a series of successes and setbacks. This process has only recently been given attention in clinical work with patients attempting habit change. Finally, the addition of Kaizen, highlighting the benefits of small steps in the direction of lifestyle goals, adds a useful element toward initiating change and "easing" patients into action rather than the abrupt shift that stage theories assume.

Chapter 7

Motivational Interviewing

Addressing Ambivalence About Change

Motivational Interviewing: Background

Motivational interviewing (MI), originally developed by William Miller and colleagues (Miller & Rollnick, 1991), was drawn from principles and techniques of multiple models of psychotherapy and health behavior. In studies of the stages of change, it became evident that patients' decisional balance changed in response to carefully worded questions. Patients progressed through the stages, not in response to directives from the therapist, but principally through reflective questions that left responsibility for change up to the patient.

While influenced by the transtheoretical model (TM), MI is distinct in that there is less concern about an individual's particular "stage" with respect to changes and greater emphasis on fluidity. The TM also implies that a patient's particular stage is relatively stable – much like a plateau – until shifts in decisional balance fairly abruptly move the individual into the next phase. MI views people as being ambivalent about change and as vacillating back and forth across various stages.

Shared Elements With Humanistic Psychotherapies

MI, while client centered, does differ somewhat from the work of Carl Rogers because it is more goal oriented and therapist directed. Therapist empathy is an important element – both for developing patient rapport and for its emphasis on personal responsibility and self-determination. In addition, while recognizing that all significant life changes occur with initial ambivalence, MI, and humanistic psychology share the assumption that individuals are striving toward greater psychological and – in the case of MI – physical health. However, rather than helping the patient to accept and integrate previously dissonant thoughts and feelings, the goal of MI is objective behavioral, rather than subjective, cognitive-affective, change.

What MI Is Not

In MI, there are no direct attempts to confront denial, refute irrational beliefs, convince, or persuade. MI recognizes that ambivalence is an ongoing, dynamic process and does not emphasize the role of education. It does, however, emphasize the role of patient values. Any information or recommendations regarding specific behavioral changes (e.g., use of nicotine patch) are delayed until the client themselves makes the case for change and is directly or indirectly asking the clinician for help in carrying out their plan.

While the psychologist may describe information about health risks, this material is not presented in a threatening, persuasive, or excessively, didactic manner but as general information. Importantly, the statements are presented as impersonal ("Many studies have found that smoking while pregnant leads to having babies that weigh less and who are in poorer general health.") rather than personal ("Because you are smoking and pregnant, you are seriously harming your unborn child.") messages. The patient is encouraged to consider the information and implicitly, apply it to themselves. For example, saying to a pregnant woman who reports binge drinking: "Women who drink while pregnant have greater risk of having a child with fetal alcohol syndrome. The alcohol damages the infant's brain while developing and these children are more likely to have mental retardation or serious learning problems. [pause] What do you think of that?" (Handmaker, Hester, & Delaney, 1999). As is evident by the last question, patients are left to interpret these factual statements and determine their relevance to their own lives.

In keeping with this approach, there are no direct attempts to confront denial, challenge irrational beliefs, or convince the patient of the need to stop engaging in health risk behavior. While deemphasizing education, MI stresses patient values and recognizes that some patient values may not be entirely rational. Any information or recommendations about techniques to assist with change (e.g., nicotine patch, 12-step meetings) are not shared until the patient has articulated their own reasons for change and directly or indirectly asks the clinician for help with the process.

Overview of the Change Process

MI recognizes that movement toward change occurs on a continuum and that the patient's cognitive and affective status plays a role in constant fluctuation across this gradient. The therapist's task is to engage the patient in reflection in a supportive manner that maintains patient autonomy. The key to change is to deliberately increase cognitive dissonance. Patients are encouraged to clearly articulate their values. Once the patient is clearly aware of issues of personal importance, they are encouraged to reflect upon how their health risk behavior (e.g., smoking and alcohol use) is consistent with or reflects those values. Some patients may explain that habits, such as excess drinking, reflect important values. ("It helps me wind down; All my friends drink – it's a big part of my social life.") Verbally reflecting these views back to the patient in an empathic tone is often powerful. Again, the motivation for change resides with the patient. In a sense, the patient talks themselves into the necessity of changing to resolve the disparity between their current lifestyle and their personal goals or desired self-image. MI includes four basic dimensions: Expression of empathy, development of discrepancy, rolling with resistance, and supporting patient self-efficacy (Miller & Rollnick, 2002). Each of these will be described in more detail.

Four Fundamental Dimensions of MI

Empathy

Genuine empathy is the relational foundation necessary for the remainder of the MI techniques. As psychologists are aware, accurate empathy includes reflection of the stated message, accompanying feelings as well as patients' felt, not yet articulated, experiences. In MI, expressions of genuine empathy will often trigger a reflection of the internal turmoil that the patient is experiencing regarding desiring to change on one hand and fearing the consequences of change and/or doubting one's ability to change on the other. It is important to recognize that much of this anxiety stems from a fear of being unsuccessful. Many patients have been telling themselves for years that they could change once their circumstances were ideal. This comforting belief will have to be abandoned if efforts to stop smoking or start exercising are unsuccessful. Patient self-efficacy, discussed further below and mentioned in the previous chapter, can help the patient see initial unsuccessful attempts as learning experiences which they can use to improve upon their efforts next time. As suggested above, change may be potentially threatening to the patient's primary relationships. This potential threat cannot be ignored and should be part of the discussion. While supporting the patient's desire to change, it is also equally important to communicate an appreciation of the difficulty of change.

If the provider experiences themselves as expressing empathy while pushing the patient toward a goal of health ("It sounds like you're worried and not really confident about your ability to succeed if you stop smoking ... but at the same time, you firmly believe you can do it."), they are moving too fast. While it is difficult not to be goal directed in these exchanges, psychologists should remember that primary care patients, in one respect, are long-term patients – they will follow up for clinic visits as specific issues arise during their life course. If their experience with the psychologist was positive and the patient experienced the clinician as genuinely understanding, they will likely return when they are ready to address their smoking, diet, or regular exercise, again. As noted in Chapter 6, clinicians should remember that most people will not succeed at the first attempt and multiple, renewed, focused efforts are necessary.

Develop Discrepancy

Patients are also encouraged to examine fundamental core values. A useful opening question is "What is (most) important to you at this point in your life?" If the client has difficulty articulating values, the provider may reflect possible values back to the patient after listening to some of their background history. For example, "It sounds like your relationship with your children is very important to you" or "It sounds like maintaining your independence is a big priority as you get older." This style of reflective listening and summarizing the patient's values may generate dissonance for the patient as they consider how smoking/heavy alcohol use/weight/sedentary lifestyle fit with personally important values and goals. Asking these questions of patients with a genuinely curious, and supportive, tone can have substantial impact. For example, the psychologist may summarize

> It sounds like you recognize the possible risks of smoking – cancer and chronic respiratory problems are two that you mentioned – but at the same time believe that you would get incredibly depressed and irritable if you stop smoking. While you were saying that you feel you've lived a good life and can accept the possibility of ill health and death, an important value is that of your grandchildren and remaining alive until they grow up. How do you put those together?

Through skilled questioning and verbal reflection, patients become aware of the inconsistency between their values and behavior. This discrepancy can only be resolved by a shift in values (not very common if commitment to them is strong) or in behavior. By continuing to be aware of the ambivalence and recognizing it, the provider maintains their alliance with the patient as they struggle with this challenge:

> While it sounds like you're not sure if you want to stop drinking, maintaining your marriage is very important to you and as you have indicated, your wife is threatening to leave if the drinking continues. While the thought of her leaving is scary, you wonder how you can manage the stress of your job without a few beers at the end of the day.

Roll With Resistance

In classical psychodynamic theory, resistance is a characteristic arising in the patient and is a way of managing anxiety about acknowledging undesirable aspects of themselves. The role of the therapist is to "break through" this resistance – typically with an interpretation of its meaning and/or repeatedly pointing out this defensive pattern. In contrast, MI views resistance as a problem in the provider-patient relationship. Within the MI paradigm, resistance is understandable since most patients are ambivalent and frequently experience opposition to self-change. Rather than being seen as a barrier to be removed, resistance simply reflects one side of the ambivalence polarity. It is also a cue that the provider has either moved too quickly to working on a concrete plan for change before the influence of ambivalence has been adequately reduced or has missed some other important aspect such as the impact of a husband's smoking cessation attempt on his still smoking spouse.

Support Self-Efficacy

Accurate expression of empathy, together with the collaborative relationship that the provider has developed with the patient, meta-communicates confidence in the patient's ability to be successful. When the provider asks patients in an inquisitive, nonjudgmental manner about the likelihood that they would be successful in behavior change, patients are typically very accurate (Miller & Rollnick, 2004). Particularly when the patient-predicted odds of success are low, the provider should pursue a discussion about possible barriers or obstacles to change. These anticipated problems should be discussed realistically. However, at the same time, the patient is encouraged to consider ways to manage these obstacles. (So it sounds like one problem that you predict will make it difficult to reduce the fat in your diet is that your wife tends to cook a lot of fried food. Any thoughts about what you could do about that?) The provider's expectations also influence patient self-efficacy. Miller and Rollnick (2004) describe a study of alcohol treatment in which patients were randomly identified as likely to be successful in recovery. Even though those patients labeled as likely to be successful were randomly selected, those patients were much more likely to be alcohol free and employed at a 1-year follow-up.

Specific MI Techniques

Asking Permission

Patients often immediately become defensive when providers plunge directly into conducting a detailed assessment or providing advice about health risk behavior. One simple, yet very powerful and effective technique is to ask the patient's permission before pursuing the topic. ("Would you mind if I ask you about your smoking?") In the few instances in which the patient indicates that they do not want to discuss the topic, their refusal should be respected. However, the fact that the question was raised and the patient indicated that it was a sensitive issue establishes that the topic is important. The psychologist can either ask permission in a later visit or recommend to the patient's primary care physician that they periodically ask the patient in the same manner at subsequent office visits. This approach to agenda setting further conveys to the patient that they are equally responsible for discussing health issues as their provider and are ultimately responsible for whether change will occur.

Asking Patients for Their Understanding of the Problem

Before providing factual information about the consequences of health issues such as smoking, drinking, and obesity, it is often helpful to ask the patient for their perspective on these conditions. In some instances, patients are genuinely unaware of risks. For example, it is still not uncommon for some women's health providers to take the position that an occasional alcoholic drink is not problematic for the developing fetus. "Advice" to this effect has been found recently in newspapers as well on the Internet. However, research has demonstrated that relatively low levels of alcohol do appear to be associated with mild cognitive difficulties in later childhood (Mengel, Searight, & Cook, 2006). The most appropriate and consistent advice is that women should not consume any alcohol during pregnancy. However, because of the wide availability of health information from an array of sources, patients may be misinformed about health risks. Similarly, a patient with a 30-year history of smoking two packs of cigarettes per day may believe that they are protected from cancer because of a parent or grandparent who had a similar smoking pattern yet lived to age 90.

As mentioned above, when misconceptions are present, providers should be careful to acknowledge that the patient's belief is not uncommon. After the appropriate information has been provided, the patient should be asked about their reaction to it. ("It sounds like what I just said is new to you. What do you think of that information?")

The Art of "Change Talk"

There are several techniques to help develop change-inducing discrepancy. First, asking the patient about their positive qualities, self-descriptions of themselves at their best, or positive characteristics that important others in their lives have mentioned, emphasize that there is more to the patient than their health risk behavior: "Can you describe yourself at your best?"; "What would you be doing?"; "What would I be seeing?"; and "What do your friends or family say about you at those times?" After summarizing these characteristics, follow-up questions ask the patient to consider how they or others see them when in pain, intoxicated, or excessively fatigued.

Asking the patient to rate themselves on a scale from 1 to 10 regarding the target behavior can be very helpful for obtaining a perspective on the importance and difficulty of change. This perspective is helpful both to the patient and to the psychologist. This technique may be used as a barometer of whether to pursue further discussion: "On a scale from 1 to 10, how interested are you in changing your diet, exercise patterns, smoking, etc.?" The patient's response opens the door to further conversation about the patient's motivation and the reality that their investment in change is often fluid rather than fixed: "You said your desire to be more active, right now, is a 5."; "How come your interest in exercising is not a 2?"; "What would it take to bring it that low?"; "How come it's not a 7?"; and "What would it take to bring it up to a 7?"

The same barometer can also be helpful in assessing self-efficacy and concretizing obstacles as well looking for conditions that would facilitate change: "On a scale from 1 to 10, what do you think the likelihood is that you will begin exercising regularly in the next month?" Once these numbers have been elicited, they can become the subject of a discussion of factors contributing to the patient's self-assessment of their ability to change. Again, the ratings can be used to highlight confidence in success as a fluctuating state rather than a fixed trait. Patients tend to view their self-confidence as a stable enduring, personality characteristic. ("I just don't have much will power.") With this new perspective, patients can begin to consider factors that would increase the likelihood of success (Rollnick, Miller, & Butler, 2008): "So, today, you see the likelihood of being able to succeed in quitting smoking as a '4.' What could bring your confidence down to a '1.' What would it take to move your confidence up to a '6'?" By beginning with factors that could reduce self-efficacy, the patient's curiosity is likely to be engaged by this unique question. Implicitly, if self-efficacy can be reduced, it is malleable and can be increased. Moreover, this line of questioning implies that many of the factors leading to a positive or negative outcome are under the patient's control.

Eliciting Values: An Average Day

The discrepancy between patient values and current behavior is the fulcrum of behavior change. In addition to eliciting values as discussed above, another technique that provides specific information is to ask the patient to summarize a typical day in their life.

> Could you take me through a typical day from the time you wake up until you go to bed. What happens, how do you feel? How does smoking fit in? If you had a magic wand and could describe an ideal day for yourself what would that be like? (Pichot, 2009).

Additional Techniques Associated With MI

As noted above, it is often necessary to present didactic information to patients. It is likely that patients in the primary care setting are more receptive to direct advice and assimilating factual content than in a more traditional psychotherapeutic relationship. A particularly useful technique in this regard is the ask-provide-ask method (Rollnick et al., 2008). Asking may take two forms. First, it may include asking the patient what they already know about the condition. It also involves asking the patient permission before presenting information. Asking permission provides the patient with a greater experience of control as well as personal responsibility for their response to the material. Saying something like "Would it be okay with you if we talked about diet?" is far less threatening and more collaborative than "I need to talk to you about your diet."

Following the patient's response, the provider can then provide factual material such as the average number of calories per day that someone of their age, gender, and body build should be consuming or that cutting down on the number of cigarettes smoked does not typically lead to cessation over the long term. These factual comments are then followed by asking the patient's reaction to the information and if they have any further questions about it.

Four principles that have been useful with MI are known by the acronym OARS (**O**pen-ended questions, **A**ffirmations, **R**eflective listening, and **S**ummarizing) (Rollnick et al., 2008). As noted above, open-ended questions ("Tell me about; Would you mind describing...") by themselves often convey empathy because the provider is expressing genuine interest in hearing the patient's perspective. Affirmations, positive statements emphasizing patient's past successes, strengths, and current motivation for change, all support self-efficacy while conveying respect for the patient's abilities. Reflective listening involves restating the patient's position in a way that conveys understanding. In addition, as noted above, these reflections may also highlight patient ambivalence. ("On one hand, you would really like to exercise because it seems to make you feel better. On the other hand, however, you are concerned about the time that it would take away from your work and family.") Finally, summarizing helps organize the patient's thinking as well as serves as a verbal platform for the next step. The summary may also be followed by a question as in the following:

> I'd like to sum up what I understand about what you've told me so far, and please jump in if I missed anything: The dental hygienist noted that your gums were swollen and bleeding during your exam and suggested that you might need surgery if you don't start taking better care of your mouth. You think that flossing is a real pain and don't see how such a minor thing can make a difference. At the same time, you want to avoid surgery at all costs. What do you make of this? (Glynn & Levensky, 2009, p. 206).

Common MI Mistakes

While psychologists are knowledgeable and skilled in patient-centered communication, the fast pace of the primary care setting can lead to making some common mistakes in applying MI. The tendency to fall into an expert mode ("It's very well known that parents who smoke at home are more likely to have children with respiratory problems including asthma.") or resort to a string of closed-ended or leading questions resembling an oral examination in which the clinician knows the correct response. ("Are you aware of the consequences of being overweight?" and "What are those consequences?") Physicians, in particular, may fall into this style of questioning because it is very common in their training to be "grilled" in a similar manner by faculty.

Rollnick et al. (2008) describe the "righting reflex" as particularly pervasive. An immediate reaction among all helping professionals is a strong urge to prevent patients from heading in harmful directions. Often our response is almost visceral and occurs impulsively. ("You can't keep drinking like that – You'll kill yourself!") In order to preserve a sense of autonomy, patients will automatically resist these powerful attempts to persuade. As the patient stakes out a position in opposition to the provider, continued attempts to persuade typically lead to the patient pulling away even more. Patients may even attempt to argue back – "Everybody in my family is overweight and they're all doing fine. Besides, I don't really see it as a big problem." Frequently, they change the subject ("Doctor, you keep talking about my diet. What I'm really having a hard time with is my stress at work. My boss just keeps piling it on and I can't keep up.") and ultimately, are less likely to return for follow-up visits.

Other common strategies likely to decrease patient motivation are those that increase fear and anxiety. Some providers believe that patient denial about the adverse effects of smoking is powerful and that a verbal assault on denial is necessary for change. Statements, such as "You're shortening your life every time you smoke a cigarette!" or "You're just continuing to damage your lungs and increase your risk for cancer," only reiterate messages that the patient has received before. Evidence indicates that while some increase in arousal does facilitate learning new information and increasing motivation, more anxiety is not necessarily better. One of the most dramatic examples of this effect are the differences in warnings required for American and Canadian cigarette packages. Rather than the customary notices describing the Surgeon General's warning that smoking is harmful to health, written warnings on Canadian cigarette packs are accompanied by very graphic photographs of cancerous growths to the lips and nose as well as pictures of blackened lungs. Despite the dramatic photographs, cigarette smoking in Canada is at approximately the same level as in the United States. Informal discussions with Canadian smokers indicate that they are aware of the message behind these photographs, but that the photographs are typically denied, ignored, or even viewed as amusing.

Because primary care visits are of short duration and sporadic, many psychologists and physicians believe that if they do not confront problem behavior now, they may not have another chance in the near future. However, a lower key approach like "You are under a lot of pressure at work. That must make it really difficult to think about things like diet and exercise. Would you mind if I asked you how you are doing with it next time we meet?" is likely to make the patient receptive to future discussions. Besides conveying empathy and support, this response, because it is so different from what the patient is used to, is particularly likely to get their attention and provoke curiosity if nothing else.

Working with the patient around realistic goals while encouraging their autonomy is a delicate issue. The significant factors associated with failure to make important lifestyle changes are unrealistic patient expectations. For behaviors such as weight loss or initiating regular exercise, patients may be influenced by the popular media – advertisements of before and after weight loss success suggest that losing over 100 pounds can be accomplished with relative ease. Unfortunately, losses of this magnitude are rare and contribute to unrealistic goal setting, subsequent failure in weight loss efforts, and a reduced likelihood of further attempts. A study of women's goals on entering a weight loss program clearly illustrates this problem. Because of the growing evidence of genetic factors in metabolism and body mass and the benefits of losing a relatively small amount of weight on cardiovascular health and diabetes risk, health authorities have established that a 5% reduction in overall body weight is an appropriate target for diet and exercise plans. However, weight loss goals set by many patients far exceed this standard. Foster and colleagues asked participants beginning a weight loss program to list out their "dream weight" (optimal weight if they could choose), "happy weight" (not an ideal weight but one that they would be happy to achieve), acceptable weight (not particularly happy with weight but could accept), disappointed weight (even though less than current weight would still be disappointed with it as an end point) (Foster, Wadden, Vogt, & Brewer, 1997). The average goal weight loss was 32.5 kg – approximately 30% of current body weight. Prior to beginning the program, participants reported that a 17% weight loss would be disappointing and a 25% loss would be acceptable but not seen as successful. The actual weight loss in the 48-week program was 16 kg – even below the disappointed weight. The average *goal* weight was three times the *actual average* weight loss. Of interest, the group reported an average of four previous diet attempts with an average of 11.5 kg lost per diet. Despite these previous experiences, participants still set unrealistic weight loss goals.

The implications of this study for weight loss self-efficacy are considerable. One of the likely reasons that patients do not remain with a weight loss program is that with unrealistic goals, patients are highly likely to rate their efforts as unsuccessful and are consequently demoralized. Therefore, in discussing this issue with patients, psychologists should provide the patients with information about realistic goals – in this example, a weight loss of 5% – and underscore the health benefits from achieving this minimal goal.

Evaluation of MI

Research on Specific MI Techniques

Empathy is the most frequently studied MI technique. A greater number of reflective statements as well as open-ended questions by the provider are associated with greater perceived empathy (Glynn & Levensky, 2009). A study of weight loss found that patients whose physicians used more empathic statements were much more likely to be committed to initiating a weight loss program (Pollak et al., 2007).

The core elements of MI, developing discrepancy and increased patient cognitive dissonance, have been less frequently examined. Miller and colleagues studied problem drinkers receiving MI versus a more traditional confrontational style of counseling. Patients whose therapists used MI exhibited twice as much-change oriented talk in sessions than those receiving a confrontational approach (Miller, Benefield, & Tonigan, 1997).

In medical settings, there is evidence that patients exhibit greater "change talk" following MI consistent statements from providers (Moyers & Martin, 2006; Moyers et al., 2007). Conversely, patients verbalize higher levels of resistance immediately following MI inconsistent statements such as the righting reflex or giving direct advice (Glynn & Levensky, 2009; Moyers & Martin, 2006). Some investigators emphasize that MI is not simply reducible to a set of techniques but is an attitude or "spirit." Indirect support for this position was summarized by Hettema, Steele, and Miller (2004) who found that manualized MI was less effective than a less prescriptive version. As Glynn and Levensky (2009) note, MI is more "a way of being" than a formula of techniques.

Supporting the concept of an "MI spirit," Pollak et al. (2007) found that patients responded better when MI concepts and techniques were included in normal physician-patient counseling. Physicians, who were not formally trained in MI, were studied in their interactions with patients regarding weight loss. When interactions contained significant elements of MI, such as affirming patient-initiated change ("It's great that you have stopped drinking sweetened tea.") or emphasizing patient responsibility for change ("Whether you lose weight is up to you.") (Pollak et al., 2007, p. 1033), patients were more likely to change their exercise patterns in the month following the encounter. Additionally, the physicians using these techniques had patients who more likely to actually begin the weight loss process. In contrast, non-MI physicians' behaviors included providing direct advice without asking permission first and demonstrating the "righting reflex" ("Well, if you want to continue on the way you are, you know your diabetes is only going to get worse.") (Pollak et al., 2007). The impact of MI in this study was particularly noteworthy given that physicians only spent an average of 7 minutes discussing weight-related topics with patients.

Global Effectiveness of MI

While MI has become extremely popular, outcome data, while supportive, are still based on a relatively small number of outcome studies. A meta-analysis of MI's effectiveness across multiple behavioral areas yielded an overall effect size of .41 (Hettema, 2007). Effect sizes were greatest for studies of diet and lowest for smoking cessation. A majority of MI studies focus on substance abuse (Dunn, Deroo, & Rivara, 2001; Rollnick et al., 2008). MI's greatest effects appear to be in getting patients into longer-term substance abuse treatment programs (Dunn et al., 2001). Similarly, there are suggestions that MI is associated with greater readiness to change – both with alcohol and heroin abusers. There is also evidence that abbreviated forms of MI may be effective. For example, Butler et al. (1999) found that relatively brief interventions (2–5 minutes) were associated with positive effects for smoking cessation. In addressing high-risk sexual behavior, MI may lead to increased condom use and decreased frequency of unprotected sex (Belcher et al., 1998; Carey et al., 1997; Dunn et al., 2001). Results are somewhat more equivocal with regard to MI's effectiveness in diet and weight loss. MI has been associated with increased exercise as well as adherence with a dietary plan but it has been difficult to establish that MI is superior to typical physician counseling in absolute weight loss (Dunn et al., 2001). While MI appears promising, a number of questions remain – among them the optimal duration of MI needed to effect meaningful change in health care settings.

Conclusion

MI is in many ways a refreshing development for behavioral health professionals who were trained that confrontation and adamant education were the only way to address health risk behaviors such as drinking and smoking. By relying on skills in which many psychologists have been well trained such as conveying empathy, reflective listening, and thoughtful open-ended questioning, MI should be a good fit for primary care counseling. While a number of brief applications of MI are being studied, the minimal level of intervention required to make enduring health behavior change is currently unknown and warrants additional investigation.

Chapter 8

Primary Care Approaches to Psychosocial Problems

BATHE and Other Brief Counseling Techniques

The BATHE Technique

BATHE is an acronym for a specific counseling protocol developed for family physicians. The BATHE technique recognizes the time limits of clinical encounters in primary care. To emphasize this, the authors (Stuart and Lieberman) titled the book describing the technique as "The Fifteen Minute Hour" which is in contrast to the 50-minute hour of traditional long-term psychotherapy. Stuart and Lieberman (2008) have trained hundreds of family physicians in the technique themselves and the approach has been readily incorporated into training programs – particularly for family physicians. Therefore, for psychologists practicing with family physicians in the United States, recently trained family doctors are likely to have been exposed to this technique. In their work with the BATHE approach, Stuart and Lieberman (2008) encouraged physicians to use this technique at every patient office visit.

Seasoned physicians can incorporate the BATHE technique while simultaneously performing parts of the physical examination. For patients who are made somewhat anxious by being examined, the BATHE technique may actually help them become more relaxed since attention is being devoted to something other than the examination itself. Other physicians will use BATHE as a fallback technique and employ it when they cannot determine any specific cause for a patient's symptoms and hypothesize that the symptoms are associated with psychosocial stressors. The BATHE technique was developed to provide a very user-friendly approach to counseling for physicians who were less comfortable in dealing with patients' psychosocial problems. In addition, it places most of the responsibility for change on the patient. The physician asks a series of questions in a particular sequence and provides a summarization of the patient's responses as well as conveys empathy. The technique is also intended to "keep things moving" so that physician and patient do not become bogged down in the details of the patient's difficulties.

Finally, because it is in a protocol-driven format with a mnemonic, it is familiar to physicians and consistent with their training in using protocols to organize sequential pieces of clinical information. It also generally assumes that patients are in some level of distress or discomfort. Because of this preexisting distress, emotional arousal is likely to be higher. With higher levels of emotionality and the presence of an authority figure, patients' suggestibility is likely to be greater. This constellation of factors reduces the likelihood that patients will oppose or resist the health care provider. The key BATHE statements are (1) **B**ackground – "What is going on in your life?"; (2) **A**ffect – "How do you feel about it?"; (3) **T**roubles – "What troubles you the most about it?"; (4) **H**andling – "How are you handling it?"; and (5) **E**mpathy – "That sounds like a very difficult situation."

Background

The most commonly used question to assess background is "What is going on in your life?" An open-ended question is deliberately used to encourage patients to describe current stressors. A major concern of physicians is that an open-ended question of this type will lead to an extended patient narrative that will far exceed the time allotted for the patient. Most research, however, does not support this concern. As noted earlier, the majority of patients, when asked an open-ended question, such as "What brings you into the office today?" will complete their narrative within 60 seconds with 90% completing the exposition within 2 minutes (Lipkin, Putnam, & Lazare, 1995). Asking more focused questions, such as "What's new" or "Is there anything particularly stressful going on in your life," or even "What would you like to talk about today," often will lead to closed-ended yes/no types of responses, which provide less useful information. Of note, research has found that physicians frequently interrupt the patient's narrative within 30 seconds. Once the patient is interrupted, they often do not have the opportunity to present additional concerns until the end of the encounter – known in primary care as the doorknob complaint. ("Doctor – before you leave, I wanted to mention these spells of crushing chest pain I've been having.") Needless to say, these encounters are extremely frustrating for physicians.

Stuart and Lieberman (2008) make the important point that the clinician does not want to encourage the patient to "tell me more about it." While this is a common request of psychotherapists, it often leads to patients and providers becoming overloaded with detail. In the BATHE interview, "less is more." Patients who are in crisis will often describe multiple stressors and details. The difficulty for the clinician is that the patient's sense of being overwhelmed may also be transmitted to them. As Yalom (1995) says in describing monopolizers in group therapy, you don't want to hear less from extremely talkative patients, you want to hear more. By this, Yalom means that the excessive flow of words and verbal rehearsal of multiple stressors actually obscure specific key elements of the patient's circumstances.

Conversely, some patients will respond to "What's going on in your life?" very minimally ("Nothing.", "OK.", "It's goin."). Cottrell (1998) suggests that these terse responses, often accompanied by deliberately averting eye contact, are more common with male patients – particularly when queried by a female clinician (Cottrell, 1998). Two responses are helpful with minimally verbal patients. First, it may be useful to briefly pause before going to the next BATHE step. Second, moving ahead by asking the patient how they feel about that – namely, that nothing seems to be going on in their lives – will often elicit engagement. ("I wish there were more going on. I'm so bored with my job I could scream!") (Stuart & Lieberman, 2008).

Affect

The clinician should keep the interview moving by asking how the patient feels about their current life situation. The affect question (How do you feel about that?) actually is very useful in moving the patient beyond rehearsal of the problem. Some patients may have difficulty detecting and articulating their affective states. Patients, particularly those with alexythymia, often will express psychological distress somatically but lack awareness of emotion. For these patients, it is often useful to "prime" them with some emotionally oriented adjectives. Saying, "Many people experiencing what you have described would feel scared or sad or angry...." This will help the emotionally constricted patient generate some feeling-oriented words as well as help them become more aware of their affective life. Stuart and Lieberman (2008) note that it is important to give patients permission to express how they feel. Many patients will see their feelings as "irrational" and may deny or minimize them. The clinician can facilitate emotional expression by emphasizing that feelings simply *are* and they may not make logical sense. Other patients will have already expressed their feelings during the "background" question. However, even if affect has been shared, it is still important to ask the "A" question directly. The answer may be very different and more enlightening the second time around.

Some patients may have difficulty moving from rehearsing the facts of the problem to describing their feelings. In these instances, it is often helpful to restate the question with greater emphasis. ("Yes, I think I understand the situation but how do you *feel* about it?") The clinician may also encounter individuals who have been indoctrinated into a worldview that intense catharsis is therapeutic ("I just need to get all my anger out!"). These patients may shout, yell, swear, and/or speak very fast. In addition to being overwhelming for the clinician, this intense free-floating affect is not helpful and is likely to be similarly overwhelming to the patient. Research has clearly shown that expressions of anger simply beget more anger. Affect, for the sake of affect, has little therapeutic value. In order for the patient to derive any benefit from their emotional experience, some associated cognitive meaning must be provided as context (Yalom & Leszcz, 2005). For the emotionally intense patient, it is likely that this pattern is long standing and, in fact, this affective volatility has actually contributed to the problem.

Troubles

The "Troubles" question – "What troubles you the most about the situation?" – begins the problem-solving process. The "troubles" component helps isolate the key aspect of a patient's distress. For example, patients that have experienced a significant life crisis often will have multiple stressors occurring simultaneously. The troubles question helps to isolate one of these issues which can then be the focus of problem solving. The question is also helpful in that many clinicians may assume that they know what is most distressing about a situation but often their assumptions are incorrect. For example, soon after the death of a parent, it is often assumed that the experience of loss and missing the deceased is the most troubling aspect. However, patients may respond that the parent's death was actually a relief since they had been suffering or that they are angry with the deceased because they have left them with a number of responsibilities such as caring for siblings or financial obligations. Even when the relationship with the deceased has been poor, there is still significant grief. As Stuart and Lieberman note, the troubles question really defines the problem. Once the problem is clearly defined, then a solution becomes much more accessible and coping skills can then be addressed.

Handling

Immediately after targeting the aspect of the problem that is most troubling, the patient should be asked how they are handling or coping with the situation. The response, while giving the clinician a rough estimate of the patient's general coping skills, will also likely suggest an intermediate solution. This step may also give the provider some clues about health issues through responses such as "I'm drinking more."; "I've upped my smoking from two to three packs a day."; "I can't stop eating even though I'm blimping out."; and "I'm yelling at my kids over stuff they can't help." If the patient does appear to be demonstrating poor coping skills, the clinician can raise a related question: "Have you thought of any other ways to cope with it?" As a general rule, when using this technique, the provider should avoid giving direct advice or suggestions. Similar to many of the counseling approaches discussed, the ultimate responsibility rests with the patient. However, if the patient does seem to be "stuck," some suggestions may be made. For example, a common recommendation that appears to improve self-efficacy as well as mood is to encourage regular physical activity. Even with patients who have been sedentary, encouraging them to walk 10–15 minutes per day if only 3–4 times per week sets the stage for an increase in exercise and often will help the patient to experience some of the benefits of regular physical activity such as improved mood and sleep. Other short-term goals include scheduling regular activities with supportive friends or beginning a journal to write about recent stressors and accompanying feelings.

Empathy

An expression of empathy concludes the encounter. While psychologists are often schooled in being able to express sensitive accurate empathy, empathy in the BATHE model is typically a verbal acknowledgment that the patient is indeed grappling with a difficult situation. The clinician conveys that they appreciate the significance of the current stressors in the patient's life.

Additional Aspects: Homework

Often the clinician and the patient develop a concrete plan for the patient to carry out before the next office visit. The plan may be relatively modest – going out to dinner with a friend in the next week. However, this assignment provides a specific task and the clinician can determine at follow-up if the task has been carried out. If the patient is being seen again in a relatively short time for a follow-up visit, the assignment is likely to be carried out so as not to disappoint the provider. If the task has not been carried out, the reasons are often more meaningful than the presence or absence of task completion. For example, a patient who reports "I was going to go to dinner with a friend as we talked about, however my mother called and insisted I spend the night with her." It is likely that relationship issues are playing a role in the patient's presenting physical or emotional concerns.

Other Aspects of BATHE

Most BATHE sessions can be conducted in 15 minutes or less. Physicians who use the technique regularly can often complete a BATHE encounter in under 5 minutes (Searight, 2007). If a complex issue is uncovered, the patient can be referred to a mental health professional. With patients being seen for a follow-up visit, the opening question should target events in the time interval from the last visit. ("What has been going on in your life since we last met?")

BATHE: Conclusion and Evidence

In general, BATHE assumes that patients have underlying strengths and competencies but are temporarily overwhelmed and cannot access these skills. The questions are designed to help patients reconnect with these strengths and reach equilibrium (Stuart & Lieberman, 2008). In addition to reestablishing the patient's previous level of functioning, BATHE may elicit psychosocial concerns that may be contributing to the patient's physical complaints or compliance with treatment. Additionally, the questions are likely to increase the patient's ability to obtain a broader perspective on current life stressors, and through the process, recognize their own problem-solving resources.

BATHE can be used as a brief screen for mood, anxiety, adjustment, and/or substance use disorders, as well as for current work or family stressors. These conditions or circumstances are important to identify because, as noted in Chapter 2, they are often the "driver" of the patient's office visit regardless of their medical condition. BATHE is also useful when patients are given an initial diagnosis of a chronic disease such as hypertension or type II diabetes. With the latter group of patients, their reactions to the questions often can illuminate possible issues with adherence or difficulties in the physician-patient relationship.

As noted above, BATHE was originally designed for family physicians who typically see a high volume of patients. A recent study found that when compared with patients who did not receive BATHE interviews, those patients whose physicians did use the technique reported greater satisfaction with aspects of their office visit (Leiblum, Schnall, Seehus, & DeMaria, 2008). Specifically, the patients receiving BATHE indicated that their physician had made a greater effort to include them in their treatment, were more satisfied with information given to them about their medication, and described better understanding of instructions for follow-up. In addition, these patients reported more satisfaction with the physician's explanation of their medical conditions, experienced being more involved in their treatment decisions, and felt that the physician was concerned about their problems (Leiblum et al., 2008).

Positive Psychology

As indicated in Chapter 4, a population-based perspective focusing on risk factor reduction can lead to quantitative health benefits on a large scale. Another approach to population health that has only recently been given attention is to improve positive coping skills. Historically, mental health, like medicine, has been focused on disease and deficit. In the past decade, beginning with the work of psychologist Martin Seligman, there has been a growing emphasis on highlighting and enhancing personal strengths (Hershberger, 2005; Seligman, 2002). This perspective, positive psychology, now has some evidence-based support. Huppert and Whittington (2003), studying a sample of over 6,000 individuals, found that mortality at 7 years was predicted more strongly by the absence of positive experiences than the presence of symptoms. Their findings are consistent with the World Health Organization's (2006) description of health as being more than simply the absence of disease. Other researchers have found that persons with a more optimistic outlook, who experience happiness more frequently and at higher levels, have better lifelong adjustment including better marital quality and longevity (Danner, Snowden, & Friesen, 2001; Peterson, Seligman, & Vaillant, 1988). Additionally, Seligman (2002) has suggested that mild to moderate levels of depressive symptoms may be effectively treated by a focus on increasing positive life experiences rather than decreasing symptomatology. Rather than focusing upon distorted interpretation and negative thought patterns as in the cognitive approach to depression, the positive psychology method attempts to sensitize patients to the meaningful and pleasant events in their daily lives.

Three Positive Psychology Interventions

Seligman has developed three techniques which are readily adaptable to the primary care context. First, patients are encouraged to document their signature strengths. In the book, *Character Strengths and Virtues*, and in the online VIA Strengths and Virtues inventory,

24 positive characteristics are listed. Examples include creativity, leadership, bravery, and spirituality. Patients can then select their own personal strengths and then are encouraged to use these strengths purposefully for 1 week and keep a log of their efforts. Research has found that this technique reduces depressive symptoms. The strengths that seem to be most strongly associated with life satisfaction include vitality, hope, gratitude, curiosity, and love (Park, Peterson, & Seligman, 2004).

Patients experiencing distress tend to neglect things that go well during the course of an average day. A simple, yet useful, technique to counter this tendency is the "three good things exercise." In this technique, the clinician asks the patient to keep a journal or diary in which, at the end of each day, they write brief accounts of three good things that have happened to them during the course of the day. In addition, the patient is asked to write a brief explanation of why each good thing occurred. By encouraging a focus on experiences for which one can be thankful in the here and now, patients are both sensitized to these experiences and can use them to refute depressinogenic cognitive distortions that everything is going wrong. Preliminary research has found that this technique also appears to increase happiness and decrease depressive symptoms several months later (Seligman, Steen, Park, & Peterson, 2005).

Finally, patients are encouraged to express gratitude to others. While this may be done through a journal or private awareness, writing a letter of gratitude to a particular person in the patient's life appears to be particularly powerful. In some instances, the patient will visit the person, read the letter to them, and leave them with a copy. Of the three approaches, gratitude appears to have the greatest enduring impact on mood and happiness.

Adapting BATHE to Positive Psychology

More recently, influenced by the positive psychology movement, Stuart and Lieberman (2008) have suggested a positive version of BATHE. In this protocol, the same acronym is used but there are some differences in the focus of questions. Stuart and Lieberman (2008) use the term "appreciative inquiry," to encourage patients to focus upon what is going well in their lives. The authors note that they originally developed this technique for family medicine faculty. They indicated that faculty meetings typically focused on departmental complaints which, in turn, led to diminished morale. Appreciative inquiry, by contrast, encouraged the faculty to highlight what was being done well and encouraged them to consider how the organization could fulfill its potential.

The BATHE mnemonic was adapted to reflect positive events and patient competencies. The positive version of BATHE is as follows: (1) **B-Best** – "What's the best thing that happened to you since I saw you last time?" (2) **A-Account** – "How do you account for that?" (3) **T-Thankfulness** – "For what are you most grateful?" (4) **H-Happen** – "How can you make things like that happen more frequently?" (5) **E-Empathy or Empowerment** – "That sounds fantastic. I believe you can do that." (Stuart & Lieberman, 2008, p. 149).

Positive BATHE may be particularly helpful for patients suffering from chronic illnesses such as kidney disease and chronic obstructive pulmonary disease. Patients with these conditions often focus upon the obstacles that the condition has created for their lives and as a result, neglect beneficial experiences. Additionally, this alternative BATHE may direct somatizing patients away from their preoccupation with physical symptoms toward other aspects of their lives. Finally, the technique can be employed when the clinician feels that the traditional BATHE has become repetitive and less meaningful to the patient (Stuart & Lieberman, 2008).

Solution-Focused Techniques

Solution-focused therapy (Nichols, 2008), while predating positive psychology, includes a similar focus on what is going right in the patient's life. However, the solution-focused approach represents a more radical departure from the medical-public health model. Rather than the traditional biomedical objective of finding the etiological factor causing illness, solution-focused therapists believe that understanding of initial causes is unnecessary. While this may seem at considerable odds with primary care practice, the solution-focused view is actually compatible with modern medicine's shift to coping with chronic disease rather than curing acute illness. Acute conditions such as a streptococcal infection, while being influenced by psychosocial factors such as stress, do have a clear definable etiology. However, conditions such as hypertension and major depressive disorder are not caused by a specific pathogen but are a final common pathway of multiple genetic, cultural, personality, biochemical, and lifestyle factors. As a result, there is no specific identifiable cause that can be identified and reversed. Solution-focused therapists believe that one does not need to know the causes of problems in order to treat them (Nichols, 2008). This approach is consistent with a positive orientation in that it assumes that patients have a number of strengths and competencies that they are unable to see because of their preoccupation with problem-saturated stories. The clinician focusing on small successes will help the patient be more aware of their competencies:

> Before giving you a prescription for the latest antidepressant, I would like to find out a bit more about your own strengths in battling depression. If you look back on the past two weeks-have there been times when you have been less depressed? When has that been and what's your explanation? What did you do that made it more tolerable? Could you do more in the future of what you felt was helpful then again? What strengths are there in your family that have seen them and you through difficult times? How do others around you manage not to get depressed? (Asen, Tomson, Young, & Tomson, 2004, p. 7).

Contributions From Narrative Therapy

Narrative therapy techniques, while having a basis in relatively complex postmodernist philosophy (Nichols, 2008), emphasize the role that language plays in generating and resolving problems. Narrative therapists argue that we live in a world that is largely constructed through communication. Language provides the building blocks of our reality.

However, this world that we construct is merely a map. Like any map, it highlights certain aspects of the external terrain and minimizes others. A topographic map highlights mountains, lakes, and rivers while a map for interstate travelers emphasizes rest stops, distance to the next service station, as well as the location of restaurants and hotels. Even though some of those restaurants and hotels may be adjacent to the beautiful lakes or majestic mountains, the travelers' map does not highlight these features. As a result, the traveler with a full bladder may not even recognize those aspects of the terrain in their urgent search for the next rest stop.

The narrative approach is helpful in that it emphasizes that all of our cognitive maps are relative and subject to revision. By highlighting certain aspects of the patient's experience and relabeling others, the patient's reality may be altered. However, with time, patients' interpretations are woven into a story with its own cause effect relationships and internal logic. These narratives, while actually just a map, have become *the territory* – the reality which determines patient beliefs, values, emotion, and behavior.

Many primary care physicians, neuropsychologists, and neurologists have seen patients diagnosed and treated for seizure disorder who have never had seizures. How does this occur? Imagine a young man, employed in a stressful, demanding, job as a forklift operator in a warehouse. One day, the patient goes to work after a particularly intense argument with his wife. When he arrives at work, the foreman yells at him in front of his fellow employees for his slow work pace. Later that day, the patient begins to have an episode of unsteadiness, dizziness, a sense of feeling overwhelmed, and being in a "fog" accompanied by physical tremulousness. The man, frightened by these physical sensations, goes to the plant's infirmary. By this time, he is very anxious and his heart is beating faster. When assessed by the company nurse, the man reports that he feels as if he is about to pass out. An ambulance is summoned and the patient is taken to the nearest hospital. In the emergency room (ER), the patient reports his symptoms. The physician asks if there is any significant health history in the man's family. The patient states that his sister was diagnosed and treated for seizures. An electroencephalogram (EEG) is performed. While the results are negative, the emergency room physician points out that the normal EEG does not necessarily rule out the possibility of seizures. The patient is instructed not to drive or operate heavy equipment until he is medically cleared to do so. Before leaving the ER, the patient is prescribed an anticonvulsant medication and referred back to his family physician for further assessment. During the ensuing week, the patient, fearing another "seizure," becomes hyperaware of any unusual physical sensations. Each time he notices tenseness in his shoulders and jaw, he begins fearing another "seizure" and immediately feels anxious and lightheaded. When following up with his family physician he describes his ER visit, his ongoing symptoms, and shows him the bottle of medication prescribed by the ER physician. Assuming that the ER physician had correctly diagnosed the patient with a seizure disorder because of the prescription and the patient's account, the family physician tells the patient not to drive and sends a note to his employer restricting work duties including driving the forklift. While the employer assigns the patient to light duty for several weeks, the plant has very few of these assignments. The patient is encouraged to go on sick leave. After being on sick leave for a period of time and being maintained on seizure medication, the patient is more convinced that they do indeed have a seizure disorder. Eventually he decides that he is unable to work and applies for disability compensation for the seizures. As is evident, once the label of "seizures" is applied, the patient's story becomes a narrative supporting the diagnosis. Many neurologists and neuropsychologists are aware of this trajectory and use caution when giving the diagnostic label, "seizure." Many prefer to use the term "nonepileptic attack disorder" rather than terms such as "seizures of unknown etiology" or "pseudo-seizures" (Rankin, Adams, & Jones, 1996).

Narrative therapists also look to the larger social and political context as forces shaping our preferred stories. For example, Epston (1994) notes that many young women in Western countries have been "recruited" into eating disorders through stories authored by the media and the fashion industry. These authorities, through magazine and television ads as well as movies, tell young women that if one is not rail-thin like many models, they are "fat." These stories are pervasive and lead to "yo-yo dieting" as well as purging through laxatives and vomiting – behaviors that are highly prevalent in the United States.

As noted earlier, direct-to-consumer marketing of pharmaceutical products also takes the form of narratives. A frequent story portrayed in television and magazine ads is that medication for erectile dysfunction will put romance back into a middle-aged marriage. Pharmacotherapy such as alopecia can improve one's social life through reversing baldness. Finally, shy consumers, anxious about speaking up at staff meetings or asking a member of the opposite sex out on a date, need only take a selective serotonin reuptake inhibitor for a natural, confident, social performance, and a more satisfying existence (Elliott, 2004). For somatosensory amplifiers, the combination of TV and Internet health news, together with a heightened sensitivity to benign physical sensations, can readily produce multiple volumes of illness stories (Barsky & Borus, 1995).

Externalizing the Problem

How Did Depression Try to Ruin Your Weekend?
Because of the malleability of language, experiences, such as anger, fear, sadness, cigarette smoking, and overeating, can be viewed in the traditional way as internal experiences over which we have no control or alternatively, and more healthily, external entities or forces that we can battle and ultimately, defeat. The primary counseling technique for changing our problem-saturated stories into more hopeful narratives is externalization. Rather than merging our identity with the problem ("I am so stressed!"), the problem is given a life of its own apart from the individual. ("If I exercise, I can keep stress away today. Stress sure got a hold of me yesterday when I ate that gallon of chocolate ice cream. I won't let stress do *that* to me again.") By changing our relationship to the problem, we can marshal our coping skills, including our social support network, in a successful counterattack. ("By keeping doughnuts out of the house, my husband can help me beat overeating.") (White, 1995).

The Value of Questions

Being in the sick role inherently involves patients bringing problem-saturated stories to the clinic. The health care system assists with authoring the stories by its focus on symptoms and further promotes the disease narrative with blood work, X-rays, throat cultures, and urinalyses. While obviously necessary, the intense problem focus has the unintended effect of preventing patients from seeing exceptions to distress. Particularly since psychological distress and nonadherence often exacerbate organic illness, intense focus on what is wrong prevents recognizing what is right in the patient's life. To "open up a new space" and begin the process of authoring a new story, patients need to be encouraged to reflect upon exceptions to their problem-saturated narratives. For a patient with depression, this process can be initiated by asking if there were any periods in the past week, if even for a short time, that depression did not enter their home or office. Unpleasant states, such as anxiety, pain, fatigue, fear, and sadness, are rarely present at the same level over time. Asking the patient about exceptions can, by itself, be effective, since it points out that they are not always depressed or in excruciating pain. It also leads to an emphasis on the problem's effects rather than focusing on its causes. This change in focus is particularly helpful for chronic illness such as lower back pain in which the cause may never be known in any absolute sense and a complete cure is unlikely. The emphasis on the effects of back pain ("What does the pain prevent you from doing that you would like to do?") leads more directly to a discussion of coping strategies rather than the continued and unprofitable search for a cure. In addition, when the patient does respond with descriptions of instances in which they were not overcome by anxiety, depression, or pain, the patient's coping skills may be highlighted by asking them what they were doing at those times. The broader implications of these brief successes can also be underscored with the question "What does it say about you that you are able to do that?" (Nichols, 2008, p. 396).

Writing as Therapy

Pennebaker (1997) has conducted a number of studies indicating that disclosing emotionally traumatic memories and experiences has a positive effect on both psychological and immunological functioning. Much of his research involves writing about past trauma and then following participants for multiple months and examining their use of health care resources. Early research found that among college students, there were fewer infirmary visits for students encouraged to write about past trauma as compared with those who wrote about a neutral event. One explanation is that the psychological and physiological demands associated with long-term inhibition of emotional reactions to stressful life events have detrimental effects. Research using immunological markers has generally supported this view (Petrie, Booth, Pennebaker, Davison, & Thomson, 1995).

Of note, the benefits from writing about trauma are qualified (Pennebaker, 1997). These qualifications are important for clinicians who recommend this technique to patients. First, there appears to be an initial period in which persons writing about traumatic events actually feel worse than those who do not engage in journaling. Fortunately, this is a brief period – usually lasting only 1–2 hours immediately afterward and at the most of 1–2 days duration. Second, consistent with the view that emotional catharsis, alone, is minimally helpful, research has found that simply writing down feelings, by itself, has reduced therapeutic value. In order to benefit from the journaling exercise, it is essential that cognitive meaning be attributed to these events. Of note, those who demonstrate improvements in health associated with journaling had used relatively few cognitive terms during the early days of journaling (Pennebaker, 1997; Pennebaker & Francis, 1996). However, later diary entries indicated that in addition to emotional expression, there was more cognitive terminology indicating meaning attributed to the experiences. One of the most dramatic studies was of middle-aged professional men who had recently lost their jobs. One half were asked to write about their experiences of getting laid off for a half hour per day for 5 days. The other half wrote about "time management" while a third group did not write at all. The results were very dramatic. At 3 months, those who wrote about their thoughts and feelings were five times as likely to have found a job than men in the other two conditions. This ratio persisted at follow-up. Pennebaker (1997) noted that the number of job interviews between groups did not differ. The major difference was that those men who had written about their experiences were more likely to be offered jobs. Pennebaker suggests that the writing process encouraged the men to "come to terms with extreme hostility" (Pennebaker, 1997, p. 39) while those who did not journal about their layoff experience continued to manifest hostility which influenced subsequent job interview performance.

Cognitive-affective journaling has been applied to patients with chronic illnesses such as HIV/AIDS, as well as in helping patients cope successfully with cancer. Postsurgical patients who have kept a journal also demonstrate improved coping skills which, in turn, appear to be associated with earlier hospital discharge (Pennebaker, 1997; Taylor, Sirois, & Tripp, 2009).

Psychologists considering this technique should ask the patient a few background questions before recommending it. Asen et al. (2004) suggest that recommending journaling to patients is similar to prescribing medication. It is important to address ambivalence and obstacles prior to making a prescriptive recommendation. A helpful place to begin is by asking the patient if they have ever done regular journaling as well as their experience of the activity. While explaining that it can be helpful, psychologists should underscore that journaling is not for everyone. If the patient does seem open to it, asking them to rate the likelihood (on a 0–100 scale) that they would actually follow through with the task on a regular basis will provide useful information. Clinicians should be aware that up to 30% of patients may have limited literacy. Because of their embarrassment and a desire to please the provider, these patients may agree to journal but are unlikely to follow through. Some useful questions that will allow them to refuse the task, while reducing embarrassment, are: "Are you the sort of person that finds it easy to write things down?" or "Some people are great at writing things down, some people are better at talking. What sort of person are you?" (Asen et al., 2004, p. 23).

Conclusion

While addressing issues such as health risk behavior and adherence are important activities for the primary care psychologist, many patients, similar to those seen in the mental health sector, will demonstrate less-specific emotional and social issues. For those patients, techniques such as BATHE, originally developed for counseling in primary care settings, as well as adaptations of therapeutic techniques developed in the managed-care era will be helpful. Positive psychology, while still in early stages, also appears to have considerable promise for addressing these problems. These techniques are all time efficient. One way to further enhance the widespread use and time savings of these techniques is to encourage homework activities such as journaling.

Chapter 9

Brief Cognitive Treatment

Problem-Solving Therapy and Acceptance and Commitment Therapy

Both of the models described in this chapter are broad-based cognitive approaches that can be used for a range of presenting problems. Problem-Solving Therapy (PST) and Acceptance and Commitment Therapy (ACT) are well-developed approaches in the mental health sector. In abbreviated forms, they are likely to be useful with primary care patients. PST is a logical stepwise process that can be applied to adherence issues, common mental health conditions, and life crises. ACT, a more recent approach, shows considerable promise as a technique for psychiatric conditions involving adverse mood states such as generalized anxiety disorder and major depressive disorder as well as for conditions associated with unremitting physical discomfort such as chronic lower back pain and tension headache.

Problem-Solving Therapy

Background

PST originated in research indicating that persons with lower levels of social competence were more likely to develop severe psychopathology. Social competence could be diminished by ongoing life stressors as well as by deficits in coping skills and problem resolution strategies. These social weaknesses contributed to difficulty responding to common life challenges, which in turn led to anxiety, anger, depression, and diminished self-worth (D'Zurilla & Nezu, 2007). The overall thrust of PST is to work with patients on a systematic approach to addressing difficulties and through these efforts teach them to use this cognitive structure to enhance their own daily coping. PST's systematic framework is useful for patients exhibiting catastrophization, a cognitive and emotional escalation process in which life difficulties are exaggerated. This ability to structure diffuse concerns and target a specific, potentially modifiable feature is particularly important when addressing psychosocial crises (Searight, 2007, 2009).

The Steps of PST

There are two fundamental phases of PST: problem orientation and problem solving (Gellis & Kenaley, 2008). Problem orientation is perhaps the most abstract part of this model. It involves helping the patient to look at psychological and physical difficulties as problems. Rather than being overwhelmed by sadness or fear, patients are taught to use these emotions as cues to the existence of a problem. This recognition should diminish the process of emotional escalation. Rather than being trapped by one's feelings, shifting to a problem-focused orientation places cognitive structure around the patient's experience and makes it manageable. By defining unpleasant emotional or physical experiences or social challenges as problems, it immediately implies that there is a solution. If the psychologist is in a setting where they have the opportunity to teach brief counseling skills to physicians, PST should be well received since physicians themselves are typically excellent, systematic, problem solvers (Robinson & Reiter, 2007; Searight, 2009).

In the next phase, patients are taught a systematic method for defining and formulating problems. First, it is necessary to break the problem down into manageable components. This phase may also include specific goals. ("I can't get along with my supervisor at work. We've been clashing for years. Lately, it just seems to be getting worse. I'm having a hard time sleeping at night and I feel apprehensive even walking into the door of the building where I work. I would like to either find a new job or find a way to continue working at my current job without being upset all the time.")

Once the problem is defined, the second step is to use brainstorming to generate alternatives. In brainstorming, individuals are encouraged to verbalize any possible solution that comes to mind no matter how outlandish or unrealistic. Sometimes, patients will have difficulty initiating a brainstorming process. The provider can start things off by suggesting some outlandish ideas. (For the patient with the difficult supervisor, the psychologist might say "You could take early retirement" or "You could ask your boss to take early retirement.") It is often helpful to write these ideas down as they are being generated. If there is a whiteboard available, this can help both the provider and patient keep track of the ideas at the same time. In examining the list of possible solutions, it is not unusual that patients' ideas center entirely upon a hope that someone else in their life will change. If this does appear to be the case, it is often helpful to refocus the patient on aspects over which they would have personal control (Searight, 2009).

In the third step, the brainstormed solutions are carefully evaluated in terms of realism. Evaluative dimensions include determining which solutions could help the patient while being minimally distressing to themselves and others. After these options are discussed, the patient is encouraged to select one or two solutions which they believe would work best for them. This process is often very freeing for patients who either catastrophize about improbable negative outcomes (Searight, 2009) or who are paralyzed into inaction by the intensity of their feelings.

Finally, the solution is implemented and results are evaluated. If obstacles arise during implementation, the patient can cycle through the steps again with this new information about barriers included in the process.

Evaluation of PST

PST has been widely studied for mental health, and more recently, for physical health conditions. Research in health care settings supports PST's efficacy with a range of clinical problems including major depressive disorder and adherence with a diabetic regimen (D'Zurilla & Nezu, 2007). A version specifically designed for primary care (PST-PC), delivered in six 30-minute sessions by nonmental health professionals, such as nurses, has been found to benefit patients with dysthymia and minor depressive disorder (Williams et al., 2000). PST-PC demonstrated clear benefits for minor depression, an enduring and disabling mood disorder, which does not respond well to medication (Oxman, Hegel, Hull, & Dietrich, 2008). PST-PC was associated with quicker improvement in symptoms compared with patients receiving usual care. In support of PST theory, Oxman et al. (2008) found that patients with a problem-avoidant coping style benefited the most from PST-PC. Shedding light on important components of PST, the process research concluded that one of the best predictors of benefiting from this strategy was the ability to understand PST's rationale and in turn, apply it early in the course of treatment (Hegel, Barrett, Cornell, & Oxman, 2002).

Robinson et al. (2008) compared PST and an antidepressant medication (escitalopram) for depression with patients recently suffering a stroke. The study was designed to determine if either treatment prevented the development of major or minor depression. Strokes are a major risk factor for both of these mood disorders with 22% and 17% of poststroke patients developing major and minor depression, respectively (Robinson et al., 2008). Both PST and medication reduced the incidence of mood disorders among these patients over a 12-month period with medication demonstrating a slight advantage (Lacasse & Leo, 2008; Robinson et al., 2008).

Meta-analyses and systematic reviews have established PST's global effectiveness with a broad range of psychiatric and medical problems. PST has consistently been demonstrated to be more effective than placebo or usual primary care but has not demonstrated greater effectiveness than other valid interventions such as medication or alternative approaches to psychotherapy (Malouff, Thorsteinsson, & Schutte, 2006). Research suggests somewhat stronger effects of PST when the problem orientation training as well as homework is part of the intervention (Malouff et al., 2006). Gellis and Kenaley (2008) concluded that the combination of PST with antidepressant medication was more effective than PST alone.

Acceptance and Commitment Therapy (ACT)

Introduction

ACT is a recent development in cognitive-behavioral treatment and is likely to have a major impact on primary care psychology in the near future. ACT is a third-generation cognitive-behavioral intervention. However, rather than a cognitive-behavioral emphasis on controlling emotions and thoughts, ACT emphasizes accepting the presence of unpleasant experiences such as physical pain, dysphoric mood, and fear, while acting in concert with one's own values (Hayes & Smith, 2005; Robinson & Reiter, 2007). A key component of ACT is the recognition that our attempts to control unpleasant experiences such as tension headaches, lower back pain, panic attacks, or social anxiety are frequently unsuccessful. Our efforts to behaviorally avoid or escape these experiences, refute irrational cognitions that are triggered by emotion, or calm autonomic turmoil, often result in our becoming hyperaware of these experiences and paradoxically increase their intensity. Furthermore, since many patients believe that these unpleasant experiences should be completely alleviated, the fact that they are continually present makes them become a singular focus of daily life. As a result, rather than carrying out meaningful day-to-day activities, the distress becomes a life-dominating experience.

Brief Overview of ACT Theory

ACT challenges Western conceptions of personality and identity. The view that a person is not their thoughts or feelings, and that these experiences can be observed in a detached manner, may be conceptually challenging for patients, and even for some mental health professionals, to grasp. ACT assumes that everyone has an observing self that maintains their core values. In addition, the observing self can readily generate behavior consistent with those values. However, this self may become fused with emotion and catastrophic thinking. When this occurs, we become focused with these distressing experiences and lose sight of what is genuinely important (i.e., our value-driven goals).

Another key construct is experiential avoidance (EA) which refers to our attempts to control thoughts and feelings. However, as noted above, efforts at control only amplify the experience. Therefore, because we are frustrated with ourselves for being depressed or because we become anxious in social situations, our reaction only makes the depression and anxiety worse (Biglan, Hayes, & Pistorello, 2008). EA has been associated with a range of outcomes including general psychological well-being, pain, and reported stress (Biglan et al., 2008). Of interest, a CO_2 gas challenge test that induced panic-like symptoms, particularly among persons predisposed to anxiety disorders, was associated with significantly lower levels of anxiety when the participants were told to accept the experience rather than avoid it (Orsillo, Roemer, Block-Lerner, LeJeune, & Herbert, 2004). Lower levels of EA have also been found to be associated with greater acceptance of pain and a willingness to carry out activities even in the presence of pain (Biglan et al., 2008).

One dramatic example of accepting painful emotional experiences comes from an interview conducted by the psychiatrist Howard Cutler with the Dalai Lama. Cutler asked the Dalai Lama about whether he had personally experienced a significant life crisis. After some reflection, the Dalai Lama responded with a story about a monk who came to him asking if he could engage in a physically rigorous spiritual practice. The Dalai Lama counseled him against the practice because of the monk's age and health. Shortly thereafter, the monk committed suicide. Cutler, taken aback by the story, asked the Dalai Lama how he got over such a terrible event. The Dalai Lama reportedly paused for a long time, apparently thinking, and finally said "I didn't get rid of it. It's still there." (Dalai Lama & Cutler, 1998).

While not as dramatic, a middle-aged man with chronic lower back pain – particularly if it is of more than a year's duration – is similarly unlikely to get completely over it. The issue becomes whether to fuse ones' identity with the experience of pain and define oneself as someone who is disabled, or live according to one's core values and accept that back pain may be an unfortunate, but not a dominating, part of one's life. From an ACT perspective, there is a distinct difference between saying "I'm in pain" and "I (the observing self) am watching the experience of pain." Trying to suppress the pain will only intensify it.

ACT in Practice

ACT is a useful model to consider with patients with chronic medical conditions, particularly chronic pain, as well as those whose are excessively sensitive to somatic sensations. ACT also shares with motivational interviewing an emphasis on patient values. While complete symptom relief is an unrealistic treatment goal for patients with these conditions, improved coping and better quality of life are possible. Therefore, a good ACT outcome is that patients are able to get on with their lives and carry out their values in the presence of unpleasant physical sensations. This lifestyle may include taking regular medication and following a diet and an exercise regimen.

In applying ACT to patients there are several guidelines. First, patients should be encouraged to reflect upon the idea of cognitive fusion with physical experiences. In addition, the clinician helps patients recognize that they have a self or identity with core values that exist apart from their illness. ("Do you believe that there is more to you than your diabetes?" "In spite of your diabetes, what is genuinely important to you?") The patient should be helped to see that when trying to live according to their own values, the lifestyle restrictions of diabetes or their chronic lower back pain will repeatedly attempt to intrude. These distractions may take the form of unpleasant and irritating, but not harmful, somatosensory experiences (dizziness, tingling sensations in the hands and feet, and fatigue) or emotional reactions to having a chronic illness and its attendant requirements. ("It's not fair that I have diabetes. It's not fair that I have to avoid eating things like chocolate and ice cream that I really love. It makes me so angry that I have to take this medicine every day.") Much like watching a film on a large screen, these experiences can be observed by the core self. However, also similar to a film, these experiences are typically brief and fleeting but do return. Through detached observation, these experiences can be separated from the core self.

However, a key contribution that ACT theorists have made to understanding chronic illness as well as somatosensory amplification is that patients expend their cognitive and emotional resources to avoid directly experiencing these unfortunate and unpleasant thoughts and feelings. For example, the observing self of the patient with type II diabetes wants to have an active life in which they are involved in church activities, physically and emotionally available to family members, and are making contributions through their work. The anxiety about the potential outcome of diabetes such as loss of sight and sensation in their limbs and the possibility of eventual amputation is realistically anxiety provoking. However, rather than observing, accepting, and tolerating this anxiety, the core self becomes distracted by anger, frustration, and the cognitive monolog of unfairness. There is an assumption in Western culture that if we have adverse health experiences, such as the diagnosis of chronic illness, the ongoing experience of unpleasant somatic sensations, or chronic lower back pain, that these dimensions become essential aspects of our being. In ACT parlance, the self fuses with these experiences with the resulting loss of direction provided by core values.

To date, nearly all of the applications of ACT to health problems involve, by primary care standards, relatively long-term therapy. Some modifications have been made that are more efficient, such as providing ACT to patients with a shared illness in a group format (Strosahl & Robinson, 2008). The personality constructs described above are likely to be particularly challenging for many patients. There have been several patient-centered workbooks that have been developed for ACT in general with particular attention to depression (Hayes & Smith, 2005) and a specific ACT application for diabetes (Gregg, Callaghan, & Hayes, 2007). Primary care patients willing to do background reading would likely benefit from brief, focused ACT.

Acceptance, Commitment, and the Physician

As Robinson and Reiter (2007) have noted, health care providers often engage in a parallel process of avoidance with chronically ill patients. For example, the middle-aged man with lower back pain for which there is no clear physical cause, continues to appear at the physician's office reporting distress. The physician, fusing with their own experiences of frustration and helplessness in the face of an implied responsibility to cure, is engaging in a form of avoidance. The physician focuses on the problem, to the exclusion of other likely psychosocial contributors, by ordering laboratory and/or radiographic studies. By ordering tests, two immediate objectives are accomplished: It may temporarily reduce the patient's distress and it reduces the physician's sense of helplessness because they are "doing something" for the patient. However, since the patient's experience is not disease, but, instead, is illness, the traditional biomedical explanatory model does not adequately explain the condition or lead to treatment. The patient, furthermore, lives in a society in which there is ready availability of medical information through both news stories as well as pharmaceutical advertisements which communicate that pain and discomfort are unnecessary and can be cured with the correct treatment ("When you eat too well – demand Di-Gel"). In the past 10 years, physicians have increasingly reported that patients arrive in their offices prediagnosed with their own plan for physician-prescribed pharmacotherapy. Again, the ubiquity of health-related ads and information about illness and its treatment provides many opportunities for fusion with physical distress and a loss of the core self.

Physicians are trained to alleviate pain and believe that symptoms must have a specific cause. Rather than accept that their patient may have life-long back pain, experiential avoidance leads the physician to recommend additional treatments including narcotics (to which many lower back pain patients become addicted), physical therapy, and eventually, surgery. Since there is no consistent association between lower back pathology and patient reports of pain (Jansen et al., 1994), these procedures are unlikely to be effective.

Psychologists aware of this pattern can be very helpful to physicians by pointing out the chronic nature of the patient's condition and explaining that despite the physician's best efforts, it is unlikely that the patient's pain, particularly if it has been present for many months, will quickly resolve. Keeping in mind the high comorbidity of chronic illness, pain, and diffuse physical symptoms, psychologists should evaluate the patient and are likely to find a treatable psychiatric condition such as major depressive disorder. However, neither the physician nor the patient should expect complete symptom alleviation. By emphasizing that this inability to cure has nothing to do with the physician's knowledge base, level of responsibility, or conscientiousness, the psychologist can help reduce this cycle. The shift in focus is illustrated by the more appropriate question to the patient: "Are you *willing* to do what would work to enhance your life and to have whatever thoughts, feelings, [or physical discomfort] arise as you do it?" The key word here is "willing" many of us do things that we have chosen even though we do not *want* to do them.

Changing the Cause-Effect Relationship

ACT's view of thoughts, feelings, and physical sensations as transient experiences with which the patient can or cannot become fused, opens a door to other therapeutic possibilities. In Chapter 2, it was noted that patients with vague somatic complaints were often not open to psychological understanding of the role of stress in their discomfort. Studies have indicated that a high percentage of these patients have major depressive disorder, which even when diagnosed, may go untreated because of concern about offending the patient with the implication of a psychiatric illness. This concern stems from the long-standing view among patients with chronic pain and somatoform disorders that their symptoms are "real" – a cause has simply not yet been found. Patients with somatoform disorders as well as those with chronic pain conditions are often unresponsive to a psychosocial understanding of their symptoms and if suggested, become clearly irritable saying that the provider does not understand: "I don't have a mental problem. There's nothing wrong with my mind! The pain is in my back. You just don't know what's causing it yet – it might be a slipped disc."

While the classic psychosomatic view holds that somatic symptoms without an organic basis are the expression of psychological distress, the alternative perspective – that physical problems cause psychological distress – is equally likely and more acceptable to the patient. In keeping with this alternative view, rather than asking the patient about the role of stress in making physical symptoms worse, it is more helpful to respect the "organic myth" (DeGood, 1983). Rather than focusing on the role of depression in causing pain, it will be more profitable to ask the patient about the role of pain in causing depression. Rather than asking "When there's more stress in your life, does your pain get worse?" or "When you have more conflict with your spouse or supervisor does it make your chest hurt more?" the clinician's questions should reverse the direction of implied causality and reflect the possibility that the pain may cause both psychiatric symptoms as well as unpleasant life circumstances: "I can really appreciate how much pain you're in. I'm wondering, does this pain ever prevent you from sleeping at night?"; "Does it wake you up in the middle of the night or does your back ever hurt so much that wake you up earlier than you need to and can't go back to sleep?" ... "I'm also wondering what effect the pain may have on your mood – You've been struggling with it for such a long time now that I wonder if it makes you feel kind of low? Does the pain ever get so bad that you don't want to eat? Does the pain prevent you from doing things in your life that you previously enjoyed?" After asking about the DSM symptoms of depression in this way, the clinician will likely find that the patient does meet criteria for major depressive disorder. However, given the patient's worldview, a psychiatric diagnosis is likely to be difficult for them to accept. As a result, the clinician should approach the patient with similar respect for their physical symptoms. As in ACT, the emphasis is on coping with physical discomfort that may not readily go away and is unlikely to be curable:

> You know Mr. Smith, you've had this back pain now for well over a year, and it really sounds like it may be making you depressed. My concern is that the back pain may not go away and we may never know exactly what is causing it. However, your doctor and I can help you cope with this pain much better so that it is not quite as disruptive of your life as it is now. Would you be interested in getting treated for depression – not to make the back pain go away but to help you cope with it better? (Searight, 1999).

Evidence Basis for ACT

While there is a reasonable amount of evidence supporting the notion that emotional avoidance is associated with a number of negative outcomes including poor health and increased pain, support for ACT as an intervention is somewhat limited. In a meta-analysis of randomized controlled ACT trials for a range of conditions, effect sizes were moderate to large in magnitude (Öst, 2008).

ACT is increasingly being used in clinical trials for common conditions encountered in primary care. In a smoking cessation study, ACT was associated with much better outcomes at 1-year follow-up for smokers. For those receiving (ACT), 35% maintained cessation versus 15% for patients receiving nicotine replacement. Consistent with ACT's philosophy of accepting adverse experiences, further evaluation indicated that those who received ACT did not experience as strong a need to avoid smoking-related thoughts and feelings to maintain cessation (Gifford, Kohlenberg, Hayes, & Antonuccio, 2004).

ACT appears to be particularly promising for improving adherence in type II diabetes. Working with low-income patients attending a public health clinic, 3 hours of ACT added to a diabetic educational group, was associated with better diabetes self-management and better blood glucose control. Similar to the smoking cessation study, acceptance of diabetes was a key factor in ACT's relative success (Biglan et al., 2008; Gregg, Callaghan, Hayes, & Glenn-Lawson, 2007).

Conclusion

Many patients respond well to a structured cognitive approach. The systematic step-by-step framework of PST may be particularly useful for patients who are emotionally overwhelmed and who benefit from structure and focus. Cognitive models should be part of the clinician's approach to patients who are in crisis. As noted above, this rational linear approach is also compatible with the reasoning process of many physicians. ACT, when implemented by skilled practitioners, does appear to be effective with a range of conditions – but particularly useful for chronic illness including pain and type II diabetes. To make ACT more user-friendly for primary care, it will be necessary to either simplify the explanatory model itself or develop a strategy for effectively teaching this model to lay people and non-mental health professionals.

Chapter 10

Cross-Cultural Issues in Primary Care Psychology

An Overview

Culture has been defined in a range of ways. However, three dimensions are consistent: (1) shared meaning and values; (2) specific patterns of social interaction; and (3) a worldview that is transmitted over time (Cohen, 2009).

Recent US population trends along with immigration patterns require that all health care professionals have knowledge of and sensitivity to the impact of diversity on illness, treatment, and interactions with the health care system. From 2000 to 2007 in the United States, the White European population grew by less than 5% while the Hispanic population grew by over 25% and the non-Hispanic, "other race" (neither African American nor White) population grew by approximately 15%. In metropolitan areas, the African American population grew twice as rapidly as that of White Europeans. As of 2007, there were 223 US counties in which non-Whites were the majority population (Rural Policy Research Institute, 2008). Presently, one out of five Americans speaks a language other than English at home (Snowden, Masland, & Guerrero, 2006).

Cultural Diversity: A Caution

As in any attempt to categorize or describe general rules for a cultural, linguistic, or religious community, a caveat is in order. There is typically greater variation within, rather than, between (a) cultural group(s) with respect to values, belief systems, models of illness, and treatment expectations. Hunt (2001) urges an attitude of humility among health care professionals:

> Culture is neither a blueprint nor an identity; individuals choose between various cultural options, and in our multicultural society, many times choose widely between the options offered by a variety of cultural traditions. It is not possible to predict the beliefs and behaviors of individuals based on their race, ethnicity, or national origin. Individuals'

group membership cannot be assumed to indicate their culture because those who share a group label may variously enact culture (Hunt, 2001).

Clinicians will benefit from maintaining a respectful openness and interest in the patients they encounter. Psychologists should also be aware of the cultural, ethnic, and spiritual-religious background that they bring to clinical work and be able to critically examine the values stemming from their own belief system.

In the early chapters of this book, a distinction was made between disease and illness. That distinction is particularly applicable in examining cross-cultural issues in health care (Kleinman, 1988). Disease reflects the biomedical perspective and deals with observable and measurable changes in the body's structure and functioning. Disease is the dominant explanatory construct of Western biomedicine. Illness, on the other hand, reflects the patient's perspective which may reflect intergenerational family views of physical dysfunction as well as culturally based etiological explanations, meaning attributed to symptoms and accepted treatments – all of which are often transmitted through the family-of-origin (Searight, 1999).

The Culture of Western Medicine

Culture, at minimum, influences, and very often, dictates explanations for the definition, cause, and expected treatment of illness. Chapters 1 and 3 describe Western medicine as a distinctive culture with its own shared meanings, norms for interpersonal interaction, and worldview to define and explain disease. Historically, medicine in the United States has reflected British and Northern European values emphasizing the primacy of cognition over emotion, a relatively exclusive definition of family (parents and their children), mechanistic science as an explanatory model, and corresponding technological and pharmaceutical intervention that addresses anatomical or physiological abnormalities (McGill & Pearce, 1996; Stein, 1982, 1993). In the United States, many patients have come to expect "high level wellness" are attuned to new interventions, and often seek more medical treatments than necessary (Coreil, 2010, p. 97).

The increased emphasis on technology and wellness as well as the consumer movement has led to a view among many sectors of the public that all diseases *are* treatable and that medical encounters should never lead to negative outcomes (Kleinman, 1988). A cursory perusal of the ads placed by personal injury attorneys support public expectations that any negative health outcome – including expected death – is a form of negligence to be addressed through litigation.

The family is actually the source of most health care. Self- and family-care include over-the-counter medications, prayer, massage, and special devices ranging from copper bracelets to humidifiers (Kleinman, 1988). Marketers of both prescription medications and complementary and alternative therapies are well aware of the emphasis on family and self-care and increasingly bypass physicians in their direct-to-patient marketing efforts (Conrad, 2007). While many practitioners think of alternative therapies as being the province of non-Western or Bohemian, antiestablishment practitioners and patients, research suggests otherwise. McGuire (1983) located over 130 "nonmedical" healing groups or individual practitioners in the largely White, middle-class suburban communities of West Essex County, New Jersey. Types of healing ranged from Pentecostal Christian groups to metaphysical organizations such as Christian Science to meditation and human potential communities such as Jain Meditation and Silva Mind Control.

Cultural Perspectives on Illness

Cultural Views of Mental Illness

Many recent immigrants are from cultures in which mental illness is equated with severe psychiatric impairment and long-term institutionalization (Gong-Guy, Cravens, & Patterson, 1990; Searight & Gafford, 2005). In these societies, receiving psychological services stigmatizes not only the recipient but their extended family and often adversely affects the marriageability of extended kin. In some Southeast Asian cultures, mental health conditions are seen as a punishment for a previous generation's transgressions (Fuji, Fukushima, & Yamamoto, 1993). Resident immigrants who are not yet US citizens may fear that a psychiatric diagnosis may lead to deportation (Gong-Guy et al., 1990).

The latest Diagnostic and Statistical Manual of Mental Disorders (DSM-IV-TR; American Psychiatric Association, 2006) includes 25 culture-bound syndromes without direct equivalents in the dominant culture. For example, "ataque de nervios," found among Hispanic women, is an episode of intense emotional expression immediately following a stressor (Oquendo, 1995). While symptoms may overlap with brief reactive psychosis, borderline personality, and panic disorder, Oquendo (1995) emphasizes that this is a culturally distinct condition characterized by time-limited expression of anger or fear. Common treatments include herbs, prayer, and spiritual counseling (Oquendo, 1995). Taijin Kyofusho, a Japanese social anxiety disorder, is characterized by a fear of offending others by ones' body odor, speech volume, or other interpersonal behavior rather than the Western fear of personal embarrassment (Kleinknecht, Dinnel, Kleinknecht, Hiruma, & Harada, 1997). Among persons of Middle Eastern and Asian background, psychological distress is often expressed with somatic symptoms such as dizziness, fatigue, lightheadedness, insomnia, and chronic back pain or headache (Gong-Guy et al., 1990; Kleinman, 1988).

Cross-Cultural Views of Physical Illness

While Western medicine has historically been founded on a separation of mind and body as well as separation of physiology from the social context, most non-Western explanations of illness are much more holistic and integrative. For example, a belief that speaking about a possible adverse outcome of illness actually makes that outcome much more real and probable, highlights the role that language and style of communication may play in physical illness apart from physiology and anatomy (Searight & Gafford, 2006). This belief is common among the Navaho in the American southwest and has been found to be one of the issues that arose when encouraging these Native American communities to develop advanced directives (Caresse & Rhodes, 1995).

Supernatural explanations of illness continue to be predominant – particularly in non-Western cultures. For example, among northern Canadian Inuit as well as the Salish, an Aboriginal community along the British Columbia coast, illness is often attributed to one's soul being lost or stolen (Grossman, Putsch, & Inui, 1993). In Latin America and the Caribbean, Susto, an experience of extreme fright, results in the soul being literally scared away. The events that can provoke Susto include observing something traumatic such as an auto accident or a sudden death of a loved one. Susto has been invoked as an explanation for a range of psychological as well as physical conditions. For example, among a group of Mexican Americans, Susto was seen as the causal factor for type II diabetes (Poss & Jezewski, 2008). Among immigrants from some Middle Eastern countries such as Iraq and Afghanistan, sudden changes in personality are attributable to a spell that has been placed on someone so that they can be manipulated by another. For example, a young Afghani woman was interested in a relationship with a young man. However, his family opposed the relationship. The woman was believed to have put a spell on her potential boyfriend so that he would have angry outbursts against his family.

Even within the realm of the body, there are other non-Western beliefs that differ considerably from mainline biomedicine. For example, the balance of hot and cold is an explanatory system used among people of a wide range of backgrounds including African American as well as Hispanic and Asian Americans. The body can be affected by hot and cold in three ways, either through physical activity and the weather or by hot and cold food. The label of "hot" or "cold" for food often has little to do with its temperature or how spicy it is. Certain foods, such as red meat, are often seen as hot foods that increase the temperature of the blood (Snow, 1993).

Eastern medicine also often focuses on the body's balance of energy. It is assumed that when there is pain or other disease there is some blockage in the circulation of vital energy. Techniques such as acupuncture and various types of massage seek to release these blockages (Erickson, 2008).

Emotion is very closely tied to illness in many cultures. It is of interest that Western medicine is beginning to recognize the role of states such as depression or chronic hostility in illness. However, indigenous cultures have a long history of including emotion as a causal factor in disease. For example, envy often leads to a casting of the "evil eye." The recipient of the force of the "evil eye" may be people, livestock, or crops. Simply by recognizing and praising them, people may fall ill if influenced by the "evil eye" (Erickson, 2008).

Among body fluids, blood is seen as having particular importance in illness and health. In some Latin American cultures, blood is seen as including the person's personality. There are narratives in Latin American folk medicine about individuals who have undergone major personality transformations as the result of receiving a blood transfusion. Among African Americans, the properties of blood often contribute to illness. For example, blood that is thick leads to slowness and lethargy. It is often necessary to "cut the blood" with fluids (Snow, 1993). One of the more common ones is pickle juice. High blood (roughly analogous to hypertension) is a condition in which the blood is unequally distributed in the body and particularly is disproportionately shunted to the upper body parts such as the face.

The emphasis on emotion and the cardiovascular system actually has empirical support. Research and social epidemiology have indicated that perceived discrimination among African Americans is associated with much greater levels of hypertension. When asked to rate overall levels of discrimination to which one has been exposed, women reporting higher levels of discrimination were twice as likely to have hypertension (Roberts, Vines, Kaufman, & James, 2007). Experimental studies have indicated that exposure to brief racist stimuli is associated with temporary increases in both systolic and diastolic blood pressure. These factors may account for the elevated levels of hypertension in the African American community with 39% of African American men and 40% of African American females currently demonstrating elevated blood pressures (Morbidity and Mortality Weekly Report, 1990). Finally, these factors appear to have long-term effects. Recent research indicates that there is a relationship between levels of residential segregation in a community and risk of death due to myocardial infarction (heart attack) among African Americans (Link & Phelan, 1995).

Treatment Expectations

Therapies typically follow from views of illness. For example, among persons of Asian background who view illness as a disturbance of hot and cold forces or humors within the body, an appropriate treatment is cupping. In cupping, small glass cups are heated and then applied at various points on the patient's body – most commonly the back. The rationale is that these hot cups will remove harmful "colds" from the body and reestablish equilibrium. Among African American patients, particularly those from the southern United States, the use of roots and other potions is a common form of treatment (Snow, 1993). These are used, in particular, when it is believed that supernatural forces or emotional factors have caused an illness. In Middle Eastern cultures, fortunetellers and other indigenous healers are often consulted to provide "counter spells" to break the hold of evil spirits. Native Americans also have specific ceremonies held by indigenous healers to cure illness.

Seeman (2008) described how Chinese immigrant women delivering babies in US hospitals have been erroneously stigmatized as neglectful mothers. During the 30 days immediately postpartum, a traditional practice, among some Chinese populations, is "doing the month," in which women are supposed to remain relatively inactive. During this period, the new mother often spends a good deal of time in bed. Exposure to strangers is discouraged during this time because of concern that they could be the source of evil spirits that could overtake the infant. Similarly, the child's name is not mentioned to outsiders because knowledge of the name would make it easier for evil spirits to enter the infant. There is great care devoted to selecting the child's name since their name is viewed as having the power to shape the child's future. Some guidelines for naming include the name, itself, having a favorable meaning; sounding pleasant when said aloud, harmonizing yin and yang, and including at least one of the central elements of Chinese medicine – metal, water, earth, fire, or wood (Seeman, 2008). During the month long period, the new mother is not to bathe or brush her teeth – she may be hand-bathed by a female relative who uses a mixture of wine and water to keep the skin from absorbing too much "wind." Cold foods, such as ice cream, fruits, and vegetables are seen as potentially harmful while hot foods such as boiled eggs and fish soup are seen as beneficial. The new mother's lack of responsiveness to outsiders, together with her reduced activity and reluctance to say the baby's name, has been misconstrued as indicating a lack of maternal attachment and possible neglect (Seeman, 2008).

Views of Western Medicine

Members of cultural groups vary in terms of the extent to which they incorporate traditional healing into Western biomedicine. Many cultures, such as East Asian patients, may use both acupuncture and formal prescription or over-the-counter medication to treat colds and chronic pain. On the other hand, there are minorities who are very suspicious of Western medicine. In the United States, probably the largest source of distrust comes from African American patients who have a history of being harmed by Western medicine and who participated in experimentation without their consent or knowledge.

Culture's Impact on Provider-Patient Interaction

As noted earlier, provider-patient language differences are becoming a major issue in medical settings. There is considerable evidence that patients with limited English proficiency receive more laboratory tests, are hospitalized for longer periods of time, and are less likely to receive preventive care (Searight & Searight, 2009). While in areas such as the US Southwest, there are a fair number of Spanish bilingual providers, many recent immigrants are from countries such as Afghanistan, Somalia, and the former Balkan states of Eastern Europe, and speak languages that are not routinely taught in US educational institutions and for which there are very few bilingual health care providers. In addition, many minorities in the United States, such as African Americans, have experienced a history of discrimination and negligence in a health care system dominated by professionals of White European background

Psychologists should recognize that nonverbal communication among members of different ethnic groups may not have similar meaning as in the predominant White European culture in the United States. Many patients who are not proficient in English may often appear to behave as if they understand what is being said to them in English and will not indicate their lack of comprehension. It is important to recognize that particularly among those from Asian backgrounds and to some extent, Latin America backgrounds, nodding the head vigorously does not necessarily mean understanding but may simply mean that the patient is trying to respectfully listen. Among East Asian Indians, shaking the head back and forth does not necessarily mean "no"; this gesture is more likely to signal that the person appreciates and understands what is being said. Eye contact, particularly between a male and a female, is often considered disrespectful in many cultures.

Because of an extended history of discrimination as well as diminished access to health care, many African American patients may view White-dominated health institutions with suspicion and distrust. Beginning in the pre-Civil War period, slaves were commonly used for medical experiments. Probably the best known example is of J. Marian Sims, a southern physician, who is considered to be the father of modern gynecology. Sims conducted experimental surgical gynecological procedures on slave women without anesthesia. Sims, generally recognized as the inventor of the hysterectomy, purchased slave women specifically for developing these procedures. The two-tiered system of segregated hospitals and health care in the United States after the Civil War through the 1960s also made many African American patients suspicious about the quality of care that they received.

Continued distrust of the health care system and the lower rates of participation in drug trial studies and organ donation among African Americans have been described as an understandable legacy of the Tuskegee Syphilis Study. This investigation, beginning in the 1920s and 1930s in the southern United States, enrolled generally poor African American males who also had low levels of education and income. These men were encouraged to participate in a longitudinal observational study of syphilis and promised free meals, medical care, and burials for their efforts. While an established treatment for syphilis, penicillin, was discovered approximately 10 years after the study began, the men in the Tuskegee Syphilis Study were never informed of the availability of treatment. The study was not stopped until the 1970s when it was uncovered by a journalist. While the exact facts of the Tuskegee Study may not be specifically known or well articulated by many patients of African American background, the suspicion that White-dominated hospitals and medical care organizations do not provide adequate care for African American patients is widespread.

Finally, an issue that has arisen in light of the American Health Insurance Portability and Accountability Act's (HIPAA) regulations and the Patient Self-Determination Act is disclosing medical "bad news" to patients. While US health care is based in an ethical and legal framework in which patients are seen as autonomous decision makers who should have all relevant information about their health, many cultures view direct disclosure of negative medical test results or directly informing patients of a serious diagnosis, to be harmful. This issue originally came to light in the early 1990s, when the Patient Self-Determination Act, with its accompanying requirements for routine discussions of advance directives and alternative decision making, was employed in some Native American health care systems.

In many cultures, it is seen as disrespectful, at minimum, and even harmful to raise the possibility of catastrophic illness or death with patients. In many Native American cultures, discussing a bad medical outcome gives it a reality and makes it more likely to happen (Caresse & Rhodes, 1995). Among other ethnic groups such as Asian Americans, it may be seen as detrimental to patients to provide them with direct information about a negative medical outcome such as cancer. In addition to being disrespectful, informing patients of a cancer diagnosis is seen as emotionally harmful – a particularly harsh disclosure at a time when a patient is already in physical distress.

In cultures in which patients are less likely to be informed directly, it is more common for family members to receive the information and to make decisions on the patient's behalf. Persons of Hispanic and Korean American background were less likely than Whites to accept that seriously ill patients should be informed of their condition and make subsequent treatment decisions (Blackhall, Murphy, Frank, Michel, & Azen, 1995). Other investigations suggest that a number of ethnic groups, including Chinese Americans (Hayslip, Hansson, Starkweather, & Dolan, 2009; Yick & Gupta, 2002) and Bosnian immigrants (Searight & Gafford, 2005), believe that family members should receive diagnostic and prognostic information and make decisions for the patient. These values appear to reflect perceptions that it is cruel and disrespectful to inform a patient of a serious illness and unduly burdensome for them to have to make treatment decisions (Blackhall et al., 1995; Searight & Gafford, 2005, 2006). This practice is seen as humanitarian and respectful rather than as paternalistic. As suggested above, African American patients in the United States are likely to desire more aggressive levels of care and are likely to be suspicious of advanced directive discussions where the issue of terminating life support and medical care at some point is raised.

In addressing these issues with patients, it has been recommended that they be asked if they would like to receive information and make decisions about their care or if they would prefer surrogate decision making (Searight & Gafford, 2006). Psychologists in health care settings are likely to encounter this culturally based pattern and are likely to be consulted when these patients' preferences are not understood by the health care staff. This communication pattern should not be interpreted as pathological denial or inappropriate family intrusiveness (Ellerby, McKenzie, McKay, Gariepy, & Kaufert, 2000; Searight & Gafford, 2005).

Practical Implications of Cross-Cultural Differences

While medical typologies of different ethnic groups are helpful in sensitizing psychologists to alternative worldviews held by their patients, it is important that these not be viewed as rigid categories. Research on advanced directives and informing patients of bad news suggests that when compared with patients of White European background, there is greater diversity in preference and opinion among patients of Korean American, African American, and Mexican American background (Blackhall et al.,1995). As noted at the outset of this chapter, in order to avoid inappropriately categorizing patients, it is important for psychologists be open to an understanding of alternative views of health and illness.

Kleinman has suggested a set of questions that are particularly useful in eliciting alternative belief systems and therapies. In particular, these questions often elicit the patient's illness narrative.

1. What do you call your problem?
2. What do you think has caused the problem?
3. Why do you think the problem began when it did?
4. What do you think the illness actually does?
5. How does the illness work?
6. Do you think that this is a short-term or long-term problem?
7. What kind of treatments or therapies do you think are necessary?
8. What types of things have you used before?
9. What are the most important results that you expect from treatment?
10. What are the chief problems that the illness has caused you?
11. What do you fear the most about the illness?

These narratives tell the story of the illness and include the meaning of the patient's symptoms within their social context (Coreil, 2010; Kleinman, 1988). When including these questions in an interview, it is important for the clinician to avoid directing the account. After the patient has completed their account, the clinician may then ask further about aspects of the narrative that were unclear. In addition, it is important to ask directly and respectfully about alternative therapies that the patient may have tried. While alternative treatment is very common in the United States with up to half of patients using alternative therapies at some point, it is unlikely that patients will volunteer this information unless specifically asked in an interested, neutral, and open manner.

Conclusion

Immigration and changing demographics are making it essential that health care professionals maintain openness to alternative worldviews of health, illness, and therapy. The dominant biomedical perspective is but one of many contemporary models employed for attributing meaning to physical and psychological distress. Patient interactions with the formal health care system, in which Western medicine predominates, often reflect an encounter between discrepant illness worldviews corresponding with differing expectations for treatment. As behavioral scientists, psychologists are likely to be particularly sensitive to culturally diverse explanations of health and illness and can be helpful in educating other health care professionals about the impact culture has on patient care.

Chapter 11

Conclusion

Putting It All Together

A Time-Focused Outline for the Primary Care Psychologist

Strosahl (2005) has developed a 30-minute format for behavioral primary care visits around which the intervention approaches that have been described can be implemented. In this structure, the initial 2–5 minutes are devoted to introducing the psychologist and patient to one another, establishing the psychologist's consulting relationship with the primary care provider, and orienting the patient to the consultation, including assessing their understanding of the reason(s) for the psychologist referral. The next 10–15 minutes are devoted to "assessment," focusing on problem definition as well as the patient's past solutions. Once the problem's parameters are clear, the remaining 5–10 minutes are devoted to a specific intervention and developing a follow-up plan. Strosahl (2005) includes 5 minutes for consultation with the physician as well as for implementing a medical treatment, such as a prescription for antidepressant medication. If the patient benefits and shows significant improvement, subsequent visits may be only 10–15 minutes in duration (Strosahl, 2005).

While this format generally assumes that most psychological interventions will be structured approaches such as problem-solving therapy (PST) or a brief discussion of acceptance and commitment therapy (ACT) supplemented by a written handout, the general format can be adapted to more open-ended approaches to counseling, such as BATHE or motivational interviewing (MI). While the visit duration may seem terribly short to most traditionally trained psychologists, these encounters are twice as long as the average primary care physician office visit in which more than one complaint would be addressed.

In choosing an intervention approach, there are several general rules to guide decision making. First, the stepped-care model suggests that the most straightforward, least intrusive, and least time-intensive approach should be implemented first. While many psychotherapists assume that patients do not respond well to direct advice, the primary care setting differs. As noted earlier, primary care physicians typically give direct advice and patients usually accept it. When the combination of the patient's physical vulnerability and emotional distress are themselves combined with the recommendations of an authority figure, adherence is more likely.

A second dimension is the type of presenting problem. For straightforward health behavior change accompanied by moderate to high levels of patient motivation, approaches such as the five "A"s and FRAMES may be sufficient. When these approaches are not well received or plans for change are not carried out, clinicians should consider models that address patient motivation more directly. These approaches would include application of the transtheoretical model, in which the focus would be on determining the patient's stage followed by a direct discussion of the pros and cons of changing. For patients with greater ambivalence about health risk behavior, MI, with exploration of patient values, will likely be more successful. For patients who have more complicated psychosocial issues or psychiatric conditions such as major depressive disorder, or who need to improve their coping skills, PST as well as ACT are indicated. Patients exhibiting broader psychosocial problems such as marital conflict or work-related stress – either with or without concurrent psychiatric conditions – can benefit from BATHE, narrative counseling approaches, and positive psychology interventions.

As the stepped care model suggests, several of these approaches may be used either sequentially or concurrently. For example, a 45-year-old male is referred to you because he would like to stop smoking. After you learn that he has been smoking approximately two packs per day for the last 15 years, you ask about his reasons for wanting to stop. He indicates that he is become increasingly aware of the health risks and also comments on the fact that he is getting older. You use the FRAMES format and ask him to note situational parameters for smoking as well as obtain frequency and duration data. He appears to be in the preparation stage and seems ready to make a quit attempt in the next several weeks. Based upon this, you recommend a stimulus control protocol in which a quit date is set, and environmental cues for smoking are eliminated (e.g., cleaning the car and home to reduce the smell of cigarette smoke, removing lighters, ashtrays, and so on, from home, work, and car) in advance of a quit date. Finally, in consultation with the patient's physician, nicotine replacement is recommended and buproprion is prescribed. Three weeks later, the patient returns indicating that he was able to maintain abstinence for 4 days but then lapsed and has been smoking fairly heavily for the past week. While normalizing the lapse as part of the change process, you ask the patient about any factors associated with the lapse. He states that approximately 24 hours after his last cigarette he began feeling irritable, sad, and tired. He indicated that his motivation was poor and also that he was having difficulty sleeping. In response to the BATHE questions, he indicates that one of the key events that triggered his smoking relapse was a conflict between the patient and his wife about disciplinary consequences for their troubled son who was suspended from school.

At this point you recognize that emotional and social factors are likely to be playing a particularly prominent role in maintaining smoking. After assessing the patient's symptoms and functioning, you recommend to the patient and his physician that he be treated with antidepressant medication. In addition, you use PST and role-playing to help the patient generate some options for addressing his son's difficulties and role-play a discussion with his wife regarding discipline. He responds well to this approach. He returns in 6 weeks with depressive symptoms much improved and a desire to try smoking cessation again. To help him get through the nicotine withdrawal period as well as to manage subsequent nicotine craving, you provide the patient with written material on ACT as well as discuss how to apply these principles to smoking cessation.

In this case, a straightforward assessment and informational approach to smoking cessation was an appropriate first-level intervention. The patient's lapse and relapse provided information about the presence of a mood disorder as well as psychosocial stressors. In addition to making nicotine withdrawal much more unpleasant, the use of smoking as a stress reliever also became apparent. This recognition led to level II interventions including treatment for depression as well as brief problem-focused counseling to address the domestic issues. If difficulties had persisted, the psychologist could have considered referring the patient – possibly with his wife – for more in-depth counseling. It is important that the primary care psychologist have a network of colleagues to whom he or she can refer when patients have a complicated clinical picture, require multiple medications, and/or have psychosocial issues likely to require more sustained treatment. Based upon the author's experience, approximately 85% of all patients seen in primary care can be effectively managed between a knowledgeable primary care psychologist and a physician. The remainder will warrant referral to an outside mental health professional for more intensive care.

The assessment phase should also include attention to cultural issues. Attitudes toward psychological intervention as well as Western medicine will be influenced by the patient's cultural background. These factors will influence what the patient perceives as being the cause of the problem as well as acceptable interventions. However, unless the patient's specific understanding is elicited and understood, the psychologist who does not consider cultural issues will be handicapped when attempting to match recommendations to patient values.

The Future of Primary Care Psychology

Primary care mental health is in its early stages and will continue to evolve. Most of the interventions described in this book, with a few exceptions, have not been well studied in their primary care application. While there is certainly support for the effectiveness of brief interventions, including evidence indicating that for some conditions brief interventions may be equally if not more effective than prolonged treatment, clear-cut evidence-based guidelines for matching interventions to presenting problems and patient characteristics are lacking.

From an historical perspective, the importance of the primary care sector for prevention, adherence, and mental health treatment has only become apparent in the past 15 years. This recognition is associated with the rise in prominence of primary care within the US health care system. Until the managed-care era of the late 1980s and early 1990s, patients could routinely go directly to specialists, and many patients had a network of specialists but did not have a primary care provider. As primary care became more central in the US health care system (Starr, 1982), the high prevalence of mental health problems, nonadherence, and the interaction of these difficulties with chronic health conditions became much more apparent. This recognition has, in turn, spurred the development of primary care psychology. However, as this book has indicated, the array and complexity of presenting problems, the necessity for consultation and collaboration, and the importance of taking a population perspective are all new to most psychologists.

Primary care is fertile territory for the development of new assessment approaches, psychotherapies, and consultation techniques within psychology. Training in this field is in its infancy. There are several postdoctoral fellowships available and primary care is included in some internships – most notably in the US Veterans Administration Health system. While there are a growing number of published resources and educational guidelines for primary care psychology, most graduate psychology programs do not have primary care tracks. Available, albeit limited, survey data suggest that there would be openings for future psychologists who have been trained for work in primary care. Of a group of family physicians surveyed, approximately 60% indicated that they would like to have an in-house psychotherapist in their office, while 13.5% already had a mental health professional providing services within their practice (Chantal, Brazeau, Rovi, Yick, & Johnson, 2005).

This book has been an attempt to provide psychologists with sufficient background information to be able to begin to navigate the culture of primary medical care. In addition, the brief, focused intervention models presented as well as the conceptual framework for integrating these approaches into a stepped care format will hopefully assist psychologists in shifting to a population-oriented practice approach. This book is an attempt to present an overview of the current state of primary care psychology. I anticipate that in the years to come, primary care mental health interventions and consultation techniques will be subjected to more rigorous evaluation so that psychologists can be guided by evidence. I also anticipate that as more psychologists enter this field alongside other health care professionals they will develop new and effective assessment and intervention techniques.

References

Aalto, M., Laine, P., Forsstrom, R., Raikaa, M., Kiviluoto, M., Seppa, K., et al. (2000). Brief intervention for female heavy drinkers in routine general practice: A 3-year randomized, controlled study. *Alcoholism, Clinical and Experimental Research, 24*(11), 1680–1686.

Allen, J. P., Reinart, D. F., & Volk, R. J. (2001). The alcohol use identification test: An aid to the recognition of alcohol problems in primary care patients. *Preventive Medicine, 33*, 428–433.

American Psychiatric Association. (2006). *The diagnostic and statistical manual of mental disorders-IV-TR*. Washington, DC: American Psychiatric Press.

Ani, C., Bazargan, M., Hindman, D., Bell, D., Rodriguez, M., & Baker, R. S. (2009). Comorbid chronic illness and the diagnosis and treatment of depression in safety net primary care settings. *Journal of the American Board of Family Practice, 22*, 123–135.

Arendt, J. T., Owens, J., Crouch, M., Stahl, J., & Carksdon, M. A. (2005). Neurobehavioral performance of residents after heavy night call vs. after heavy alcohol ingestion. *Journal of the American Medical Association, 294*, 1025–1033.

Armitage, C. J. (2008). A volitional help sheet to encourage smoking cessation: A randomized exploratory trial. *Health Psychology, 27*(5), 557–566.

Asen, E., Tomson, D., Young, V., & Tomson, P. (2004). *Ten minutes for the family: Systemic practice in primary care*. London: Routledge.

Babor, T. F., Aguirre-Molina, M., Marlatt, G. A., & Clayton, R. (1999). Managing alcohol problems and risky drinking. *American Journal of Health Promotion, 14*, 98–103.

Bailey, K. A., Chavira, D. A., Stein, M. T., & Stein, M. B. (2006). Brief measures to screen for social phobia in primary care pediatrics. *Journal of Pediatric Psychology, 31*(5), 512–521.

Bair, M. J., Robinson, R. L., Katon, W., & Kroenke, K. (2003). Depression and pain comorbidity: A literature review. *Archives of Internal Medicine, 163*, 2433–2445.

Balint, M. (1964). *The doctor, his patient, and the illness*. London: Pitman Medical.

Ballesteros, J., Gonzalez-Pinto, A., Querejeta, I., & Arino, J. (2004). Brief interventions for hazardous drinkers delivered in primary care are equally effective for men and women. *Addiction, 99*, 103–108.

Barrett, J. E., Barrett, J. A., Oxman, T. E., & Gerber, P. D. (1988). The prevalence of psychiatric disorders in a primary care practice. *Archives of General Psychiatry, 45*, 1100–1106.

Barsky, A. J., & Borus, J. F. (1995). Somatization and medicalization in the era of managed care. *Journal of the American Medical Association, 274*, 1931–1934.

Beck, A. T., & Steer, R. A. (1993). *Beck depression inventory manual*. New York: Psychological Corporation.

Beck, A. T., Steer, R. A., Ball, R., Ciervo, C. A., & Kabat, M. (1997). Use of the Beck anxiety and depression inventories for primary care with medical outpatients. *Assessment, 4*, 211–219.

Beck, A. T., Steer, R. A., & Brown, G. K. (1996). *Manual for the Beck depression inventory-II*. San Antonio: Psychological Corporation.

Beekman, A. T. F., Deeg, D. J. H., Braaam, A. W., Smit, J. H., & Van Tilberg, W. (1997). Consequences of major and minor depression in later life: A study of disability, well-being and service utilization. *Psychological Medicine, 27*, 1397–1409.

Belcher, L., Kalichman, S., Topping, M., Smith, S., Emshoff, J., Norris, F., et al. (1998). A randomized trial of a brief HIV risk reduction counseling intervention for women. *Journal of Consulting and Clinical Psychology, 66*, 531–541.

Berkman, L. K. (2004). *Social epidemiology*. New York: Oxford.

Berner, C., Gunzler, C., Frick, K., Kriston, L., Loessl, B., Bruck, R., et al. (2008). Finding the ideal place for a psychotherapeutic intervention in a stepped care approach – A brief overview of the literature and preliminary results from the project predict. *International Journal of Methods in Psychiatric Research, 17*(S1), S60–S64.

Biglan, A., Hayes, S. C., & Pistorello, J. (2008). Acceptance and commitment: Implications for prevention science. *Prevention Science, 9*, 139–152.

Blackhall, L. J., Murphy, S. T., Frank, G., Michel, V., & Azen, S. (1995). Ethnicity and attitudes towards patient autonomy. *Journal of the American Medical Association, 274*, 820–825.

Bor, R., & McCann, D. (1999). Introduction. In R. Bor & D. McCann (Eds.), *The practice of counseling in primary care*. London: Sage.

Bower, P., Rowland, N., & Hardy, R. (2003). The clinical effectiveness of counseling in primary care: A systematic review and meta-analysis. *Psychological Medicine, 33*, 203–215.

Bray, J. H., Frank, R. G., McDaniel, S. H., & Heldring, M. (2004). Education, practice, and research opportunities for psychologists in primary care. In R. G. Frank, S. H. McDaniel, J. H. Bray, & M. Heldring (Eds.), *Primary care psychology* (pp. 3–22). Washington, DC: American Psychological Association.

Brody, D. S., Khaliq, A. A., & Thompson, T. L. (1997). Patients' perspectives of the management of emotional distress in primary care settings. *Journal of General Internal Medicine, 12*, 403–406.

Brugha, T. S. (2002). The end of the beginning: A requiem for the categorization of mental disorder. *Psychological Medicine, 32*, 1149–1154.

Butler, C. C., Rollnick, S., Cohen, D., Russel, I., Bachman, M., & Stott, N. (1999). Motivational consulting versus brief advice for smokers in general practice: A randomised trial. *British Journal of General Practice, 49*, 611–616.

Canadian Society for Exercise Physiology. (1994). *Physical Activity Readiness Questionnaire*. Ottawa: Health Canada.

Cano, A., Sprafkin, R. P., Scaturo, D. J., Lantinga, L. J., Fiese, B. H., & Brand, F. (2001). Mental health screening in primary care: A comparison of 3 brief measures of psychological distress. *Primary Care Companion to the Journal of Clinical Psychiatry, 3*(5), 206–210.

Caplan, G., & Caplan, R. B. (1993). *Mental health consultation and collaboration*. San Francisco: Jossey-Bass.

Caresse, J. A., & Rhodes, L. A. (1995). Western bioethics on the Navajo reservation, benefit or harm? *Journal of the American Medical Association, 274*, 826–829.

Carey, M. P., Maisto, S. A., Kalichman, S. C., Forsyth, A. D., Wright, E. M., & Johnson, B. (1997). Enhancing motivation to reduce the risk of HIV infection for economically disadvantaged urban women. *Journal of Consulting and Clinical Psychology, 65*, 531–541.

Carey, T. A., & Mullan, R. J. (2007). Patients taking the lead. A naturalistic investigation of a patient led approach to treatment in primary care. *Counselling Psychology Quarterly, 20*(1), 27–40.

Cassell, E. J. (1997). *Doctoring: The nature of primary care medicine*. New York: Oxford University Press.

Centers for Disease Control. (1990). Topics in minority health: Health beliefs and compliance with prescribed medication for hypertension among black women – New Orleans, 1985-86. *Morbidity and Mortality Weekly Report, 39*(40), 701–704.

Centers for Disease Control. (2005). QuickStats: Percentage of adults aged >18 years who used complementary and alternative medicine (CAM) during the preceding 12 months, by sex – United States, 2002. *Morbidity and Mortality Weekly Report, 54*(11), 283.

Champion, V. L., & Skinner, C. S. (2008). The health belief model. In K. Glanz, B. K. Rimer, & K. Viswanath (Eds.), *Health behavior and health education*. San Francisco: Jossey-Bass.

Chang, G., Goetz, M. A., Wilkins-Haug, L., & Berman, S. (1999). Identifying prenatal alcohol use: Screening instruments versus clinical predictors. *American Journal on Addictions, 8*, 87–93.

Chantal, M. L. R., Brazeau, C. M., Rovi, S., Yick, C., & Johnson, M. S. (2005). Collaboration between mental health professionals and family physicians: A survey of New Jersey family physicians. *Primary Care Companion to the Journal of Clinical Psychiatry, 7*, 12–14.

Cherry, N. (1976). Persistent job changing: Is it a problem? *Journal of Occupational Psychology, 49*, 203–221.

Christensen, H., Griffiths, K. M., Mackinnon, A. J., & Britliffe, K. (2006). Online randomized controlled trial of brief and full cognitive behaviour therapy for depression. *Psychological Medicine, 36*, 1737–1746.

Cohen, A. B. (2009). Many forms of culture. *American Psychologist, 64*(3), 194–204.

Collins, R. L. (2005). Relapse prevention for eating disorders and obesity. In G. A. Marlatt & M. Donovan (Eds.), *Relapse prevention: Maintenance strategies in the treatment of addictive behaviors* (pp. 248–275). New York: Guilford.

Comer, R. J. (2010). *Abnormal psychology* (7th ed.). New York: Worth.

Connors, C. J., & Stewart, S. H. (2004). Alcohol and other substance use disorders. In L. Haas (Ed.), *Handbook of primary care psychology* (pp. 187–200). New York: Oxford.

Conrad, P. (2007). *The medicalization of society*. Baltimore, MD: Johns Hopkins University Press.

Coreil, J. (2010). Social epidemiology. In J. Coreil (Ed.), *Social and behavioral foundations of public health* (pp. 45–65). Thousand Oaks, CA: Sage.

Cottrell, K. (1998). Psychiatric technique may help time strapped FPs. *Canadian Medical Association Journal, 159*(7), 753.

Coyne, J. C., Thompson, R., Palmer, S. C., & Kagee, A. (2000). Should we screen for depression? Caveats and potential pitfalls. *Applied and Preventive Psychology, 9*, 101–121.

Crum, R. M., Anthony, J. C., Bassett, S. S., & Folstein, M. F. (1993). Population-based norms for the Mini-Mental State Examination by age and educational level. *Journal of the American Medical Association, 269*, 2386–2391.

Cummings, N. A., O'Donohue, W., Hayes, S. C., & Follette, V. (2001). *Integrated behavioral healthcare*. San Diego, CA: Academic Press.

Currie, S., & Wang, J. (2004). Chronic pain and major depression in the general Canadian population. *Pain, 107*, 54–60.

Cwikel, J., Zilber, N., Feinson, M., & Lerner, Y. (2008). Prevalence and risk factors of threshold and subthreshold psychiatric disorders in primary care. *Social Psychiatry and Social Epidemiology, 43*, 184–191.

Dalai Lama., & Cutler, H. C. (1998). *The art of happiness*. New York: Riverhead Books.

Danner, D., Snowden, D., & Friesen, W. (2001). Positive emotions in early life and longevity. *Journal of Personality and Social Psychology, 80*, 804–813.

Davy, J. (1999). A biopsychosocial approach to counseling in primary care. In R. Bor & D. McCann (Eds.), *The practice of primary care counseling* (pp. 24–41). London: Sage.

DeGood, D. E. (1983). Reducing medical patients' reluctance to participate in psychological therapies: The initial session. *Professional Psychology: Research and Practice, 14*, 570–579.

Denollet, J., Maas, K., Knottnerus, A., Keyzer, J. J., & Pop, V. (2009). Anxiety predicted premature all-cause and cardiovascular death in a 10 year follow-up of middle-aged women. *Journal of Clinical Epidemiology, 62*, 452–456.

D'Eramo-Melkus, G., & Demas, P. (1989). Patient perceptions of diabetic treatment goals. *Diabetes Educator, 15*, 440–443.

Derogatis, L. R., Lipman, R. S., & Covi, L. (1973). The SCL-90: An outpatient psychiatric rating scale. *Psychopharmacology Bulletin, 9*, 13–28.

DiClemente, C. C., Prochaska, J. O., Fairhurst, S. K., Velcier, W. F., Velasquez, M. M., & Rossi, J. S. (1991). The process of smoking cessation: An analysis of precontemplation, contemplation, and preparation stages of change. *Journal of Consulting and Clinical Psychology, 59*, 295–304.

DiMatteo, M. R. (2004). Variations in patients' adherence to medical recommendations: A quantitative review of 50 years of research. *Medical Care, 42*(2), 200–209.

D'Onofrio, G., & Degutis, L. C. (2004). Screening and brief intervention in the emergency department. *Alcohol Research & Health, 28*(2), 63–72.

Dunn, C., Deroo, L., & Rivara, F. P. (2001). The use of brief interventions adapted from motivational interviewing. *Addiction, 96*, 1725–1742.

D'Zurilla, T. J., & Nezu, A. M. (2007). *Problem-solving therapy: A positive approach to clinical intervention* (3rd ed.). New York: Springer.

Ellerby, J. H., McKenzie, J., McKay, S., Gariepy, G. J., & Kaufert, J. M. (2000). Bioethics for clinicians: Aboriginal cultures. *Canadian Medical Association Journal, 163*(7), 845–850.

Elliott, C. (2004). *Better than well: American medicine meets the American dream.* New York: Norton.

Epstein, R. M., Quill, T. E., & McWhiney, I. R. (1999). Somatization reconsidered: Incorporating the patient's experience of illness. *Archives of Internal Medicine, 159*, 215–222.

Epston, D. (1994). Extending the conversation. *Family Therapy Networker, 18*, 30–37, 62.

Erickson, P. I. (2008). *Ethnomedicine.* Long Grove, IL: Waveland Press.

Fallon, B., Kochevar, J., Gaito, A., & Nields, J. A. (1998). The underdiagnosis of neuropsychiatric Lyme disease in children and adults. *Psychiatric Clinics of North America, 21*, 693–703.

Fiore, M. C., Bailey, W. C., Cohen, S. J., Dorfman, S. F., Goldstein, M. G., Gritz, E. R., et al. (2000). *Treating tobacco use and dependence.* Washington, DC: US Department of Health and Human Services.

Fleming, M. F., Manwell, L. B., Barry, K. L., & Johnson, K. (1998). At-risk drinking in an HMO primary care sample: Prevalence and health policy implications. *American Journal of Public Health, 88*(1), 90–93.

Folstein, M. F., Folstein, S. E., & McHugh, P. R. (1975). "Mini mental state:" A practical method for grading the cognitive state of patients for the clinician. *The Journal of Psychiatric Research, 12*, 189–198.

Foster, G. D., Wadden, T. A., Vogt, R. A., & Brewer, G. (1997). What is a reasonable weight loss? Patients' expectations and evaluations of obesity treatment outcomes. *Journal of Consulting and Clinical Psychology, 65*(1), 79–85.

Freedman, M., Leach, L., Kaplan, E., Winocur, G., Shulman, K. I., & Delis, D. (1994). *Clock drawing: A neuropsychological analysis.* New York: Oxford University Press.

Fuji, J. S., Fukushima, S. N., & Yamamoto, J. (1993). Psychiatric care of Japanese-Americans. In A. C. Gaw (Ed.), *Culture, ethnicity and mental illness* (pp. 305–346). Washington, DC: American Psychiatric Press.

Future of Family Medicine Project Leadership Committee. (2004). The future of family medicine: A collaborative project of the family medicine community. *Annals of Family Medicine, 2*, S3–S32, doi: 10.1370/afm.130.

Gellis, Z. D., & Kenaley, B. (2008). Problem-solving therapy for depression in adults: A systematic review. *Research on Social Work Practice, 18*, 117–131.

Gifford, E. V., Kohlenberg, B. S., Hayes, S. C., & Antonuccio, D. O. (2004). Acceptance-based treatment for smoking cessation. *Behavior Therapy, 35*, 689–705.

Gilchrist, V. J., Stange, K. C., Flocke, S. A., McCord, G., & Bourguet, C. (2004). A comparison of the National Ambulatory Care Survey (NAMCS) measurement approach with direct observation of outpatient visits. *Medical Care, 42*, 276–280.

Glynn, L. H., & Levensky, E. R. (2009). Promoting treatment adherence using motivational interviewing: Guidelines and tools. In L. C. James & W. T. O'Donohue (Eds.), *The primary care toolkit* (pp. 199–210). New York: Springer.

Goldberg, D., Bridges, K., Duncan-Jones, P., & Grayson, D. (1988). Detecting anxiety and depression in general medical settings. *British Medical Journal, 297*, 897–899.

Goldberg, D. P., & Williams, P. (1988). *A user's guide to the GHQ.* Windsor: NFER-Nelson.

Goldstein, J. (1990). Desperately seeking science: The creation of knowledge in family practice. *Hastings Center Report, 20*(6), 26–32.

Gong-Guy, E., Cravens, R. B., & Patterson, T. E. (1990). Clinical issues in mental health service delivery to refugees. *American Psychologist, 46,* 642–648.

Gregg, J. A., Callaghan, G. M., & Hayes, S. C. (2007). *The diabetes lifestyle book.* Oakland, CA: New Harbringer.

Gregg, J. A., Callaghan, G. M., Hayes, S. C., & Glenn-Lawson, J. L. (2007). Improving diabetes self-management through acceptance, mindfulness, and values: A randomized controlled trial. *Journal of Consulting and Clinical Psychology, 75*(2), 336–343.

Groopman, J. (2007). *How doctors think.* Boston: Houghton Mifflin.

Grossman, D. C., Putsch, R. W., & Inui, T. S. (1993). The meaning of death in an American Indian community. *Family Medicine, 25,* 593–597.

Guerrero, A. (2003). General medical considerations in child and adolescent patients who present with psychiatric symptoms. *Child and Adolescent Psychiatric Clinics of North America, 12,* 613–628.

Hamilton, M. (1967). Development of a rating scale for primary depressive illness. *British Journal of Social and Clinical Psychology, 6,* 278–296.

Handmaker, N. S., Hester, R. K., & Delaney, H. D. (1999). *Motivating pregnant women to stop drinking (videotape).* Behavior Therapy Associates.

Hayes, S. C., & Smith, S. (2005). *Get out of your mind and into your life.* Oakland, CA: New Harbringer.

Hayslip, B., Hansson, R. O., Starkweater, J. D., & Dolan, D. C. (2009). Culture, individual diversity, and end-of-life decisions. In J. L. Werth & D. Blevins (Eds.), *Decision making near the end of life* (pp. 301–324). New York: Routledge.

He, Y., Lin, E. H. B., Bruffaerts, R., Posada-Villa, J., Angemeyer, M. C., Levinson, D., et al. (2008). Mental disorders among persons with arthritis: Results from the World Mental Health Surveys. *Psychological Medicine, 38,* 1639–1650.

Heatherton, T. F., Kozlowski, L. T., Frecker, K. O., & Fagerstrom, K. (1991). The Fagerstrom test for nicotine dependence: A revision of the Fagerstrom Tolerance Questionnaire. *British Journal of Addiction, 86,* 1119–1127.

Hegel, M. T., Barrett, J. E., Cornell, J. E., & Oxman, T. E. (2002). Predictors of response to problem-solving treatment of depression in primary care. *Behavior Therapy, 33*(4), 511–527.

Hershberger, P. J. (2005). Prescribing happiness: Positive psychology and family medicine. *Family Medicine, 37*(9), 630–634.

Herzig, K., Huynh, D., Gilbert, P., Danley, D. W., Jackson, R., & Gerbert, B. (2006). Comparing prenatal providers' approaches to four different risks: Alcohol, tobacco, drugs and domestic violence. *Women & Health, 43*(3), 83–101.

Hettema, J. E. (2007). *A meta-analysis of motivational interviewing across behavioral domains.* Albuquerque, New Mexico: University of New Mexico (dissertation).

Hettema, J., Steele, J., & Miller, W. R. (2005). Motivational interviewing. *Annual Review of Clinical Psychology, 1,* 91–111.

Hirschfeld, R. M. A., Williams, J. B. W., Spitzer, R. L., Calabrese, J. R., Flynn, L., Keck, P. E., et al. (2000). Development and validation of a screening instrument for bipolar spectrum disorder. *American Journal of Psychiatry, 157,* 1873–1875.

Hooley, J. M., & Teasdale, J. D. (1989). Predictors of relapse in unipolar depression: Expressed emotion, marital distress and perceived criticism. *Journal of Abnormal Psychology, 98,* 229–235.

Hunter, C. L., Goodie, J. L., Oordt, M. S., & Dobmeyer, A. C. (2009). *Integrated behavioral health in primary care.* Washington, DC: American Psychological Association.

Huppert, F. A. (2009). A new approach to reducing disorder and improving well-being. *Perspectives on Psychological Science, 4*(1), 108–111.

Huppert, F. A., Johnson, T., & Nickson, J. (2000). High prevalence of prospective memory impairment in the elderly and in early-stage dementia: Findings from a population-based study. *Applied Cognitive Psychology, 14,* S63–S81.

Huppert, F. A., & Whittington, J. E. (2003). Evidence for the independence of positive and negative well-being: Implications for quality of life assessment. *British Journal of Health Psychology, 8,* 107–119.

Italian Collaborative Group for the Study of Psychopathological Factors in Primary Headache. (2002). Psychiatric comorbidity and psychosocial stress in patients with tension-type headache from headache centers in Italy. *Cephalalgia, 19,* 159–164.

Jacobson, N. S., Dobson, K., Fruzzetti, A. E., Schmaling, K. B., & Salusky, S. (1991). Marital therapy as a treatment for depression. *Journal of Consulting and Clinical Psychology, 59,* 347–357.

Jansen, M. C., Brant-Zawadzki, M. N., Obuchowski, N., Modic, M. T., Malkasian, D., & Ross, J. S. (1994). Magnetic resonance imaging of the lumbar spine in people without back pain. *New England Journal of Medicine, 331,* 69–73.

Johnson, S. K. (2008). *Medically unexplained illness: Gender and biopsychosocial implications.* Washington, DC: American Psychological Association.

Johnson, S. S., Paiva, A. L., Cummins, C. O., Johnson, J. L., Dymet, S. J., Wright, J. A., et al. (2007). Transtheoretical-model based multiple behavior intervention for weight management: Effectiveness on a population basis. *Preventive Medicine, 46,* 238–246.

Juang, K., Wang, S., Fuh, J., Lu, S., & Su, T. (2000). Comorbidity of depressive and anxiety disorders in chronic daily headache and its subtypes. *Headache: The Journal of Head and Face Pain, 10,* 818–823.

Katon, W. J. (2003). Clinical and health services relationships between major depression, depressive symptoms, and general medical illness. *Biological Psychiatry, 54,* 216–226.

Katz, D. L. (2001). Behavior modification in primary care: The pressure system model. *Preventive Medicine, 32,* 66–72.

Kendler, K. S., Neale, M. C., Kessler, R. C., Heath, A. C., & Eaves, L. J. (1993). Panic disorder in women: A population-based twin study. *Psychological Medicine, 23,* 397–406.

Kessler, R. C., Chiu, W. T., Demler, O., & Walters, E. E. (2005). Prevalence, severity, and comorbidity of 12 month DSM-IV disorders in the national comorbidity survey replication. *Archives of General Psychiatry, 62,* 617–627.

Kleinknecht, R. A., Dinnel, D. L., Kleinknecht, E. E., Hiruma, N., & Harada, N. (1997). Cultural factors in social anxiety: A comparison of social phobia symptoms and Taijin Kyofusho. *Journal of Anxiety Disorders, 11,* 157–177.

Kleinman, A. (1988). *The illness narratives: Suffering, healing and the human condition.* New York: Basic Books.

Kroenke, K., & Mangelsdorf, A. D. (1989). Common symptoms in ambulatory care: Incidence, evaluation, therapy, and outcome. *American Journal of Medicine, 86,* 262–266.

Kroenke, K., Spitzer, R. L., Williams, J. B. W., Monahan, P. O., & Lowe, B. (2007). Anxiety disorders in primary care: Prevalence, impairment, comorbidity, and detection. *Annals of Internal Medicine, 146*(5), 317–325.

Kush, F. R. (2001). Primary care and clinical psychology: Assessment strategies in medical settings. *Journal of Clinical Psychology in Medical Settings, 8,* 219–228.

Lacasse, J. L., & Leo, J. (2008). Escitalopram, problem-solving therapy, and poststroke depression. *Journal of the American Medical Association, 300,* 1757–1758.

Leiblum, S. R., Schnall, E., Seehus, M., & DeMaria, A. (2008). To BATHE or not to BATHE: Patient satisfaction with visits to their family physician. *Family Medicine, 40*(6), 407–411.

Lin, E. H. B., Katon, W., Von Korff, M., Tang, L., Williams, J. W., Kroenke, K., et al. (2003). Effect of improving depression care on pain and functional outcomes among older adults with arthritis: A randomized controlled trial. *Journal of the American Medical Association, 290,* 2428–2434.

Link, B. P., & Phelan, J. (1995). Social conditions as fundamental causes of illness. *Journal of Health and Social Behavior,* 80–94.

Linton, J. C. (2004). Psychological assessment in primary care. In L. Haas (Ed.), *Handbook of primary care psychology* (pp. 35–46). New York: Oxford.

Lipkin, M., Putnam, S., & Lazare, A. (1995). *The medical interview.* New York: Springer.

Lyness, J. M., Chapman, B. P., McGriff, J., Drayer, R., & Duberstein, P. R. (2008). One year outcomes in minor and subsyndromal depression in older primary care patients. *International Psychogeriatrics, 21*(1), 60–68.

Lyness, J. M., Heo, M., Datto, C. J., Ten Have, T. R., Katz, I. R., Drayer, R., et al. (2006). Outcomes of minor and subsyndromal depression among elderly patients in primary care settings. *Annals of Internal Medicine, 144,* 496–504.

Malla, A., & Merskey, H. (1987). Screening for alcoholism in family practice. *Family Practice Research Journal, 6,* 138–147.

Malouff, J. M., Thorsteinsson, E. B., & Schutte, N. S. (2006). The efficacy of problem solving therapy in reducing mental and physical health problems: A meta-analysis. *Clinical Psychology Review, 27,* 46–57.

Marlatt, G. A., & Donovan, D. M. (2005). *Relapse prevention* (2nd ed.). New York: Guilford.

Marlatt, G. A., & Witkiewitz, K. (2005). Relapse prevention for alcohol and drug problems. In G. A. Marlatt & K. Witkiewitz (Eds.), *Relapse prevention* (2nd ed.). New York: Guilford.

Maurer, R. (2004). *One small step can change your life.* New York: Workman Publishing.

May, H. T., Horne, B. D., Carlquist, J. F., Sheng, X., Joy, E., & Catinella, A. P. (2009). Depression after coronary artery disease is associated with heart failure. *Journal of the American College of Cardiology, 53,* 1440–1447.

Mayes, R., Bagwell, C., & Erkulwater, J. L. (2009). *Medicating children: AD/HD and pediatric mental health.* Cambridge, MA: Harvard University Press.

Mayfield, D., McCleod, G., & Hall, P. (1974). The CAGE questionnaire: Validation of a new alcoholism screening instrument. *American Journal of Psychiatry, 131,* 1121–1123.

McGill, D. W., & Pearce, J. K. (1996). American families with English ancestors from the Colonial era: Anglo Americans. In M. McGoldrick, J. Giordano & J. K. Pearce (Eds.), *Ethnicity and family therapy* (2nd ed., pp. 451–466). New York: Guilford.

McGuire, M. B. (1983). Words of power: Personal empowerment and healing. *Culture, Medicine, and Psychiatry, 7,* 221–240.

Mengel, M., & Schwiebert, P. (2009). *Family medicine: Ambulatory care and prevention.* New York: McGraw-Hill.

Mengel, M. B., Searight, H. R., & Cook, K. (2006). Preventing alcohol-exposed pregnancies. *Journal of the American Board of Family Medicine, 19*(5), 494–505.

Miller, W. L. (1992). Routine, ceremony, or drama: An exploratory study of the primary care clinical encounter. *Journal of Family Practice, 34*(3), 289–298.

Miller, W. R., Benefield, R. S., & Tonigan, J. S. (1997). Enhancing motivation for change in problem drinking: A controlled comparison of two therapist styles. *Journal of Consulting and Clinical Psychology, 61,* 455–461.

Miller, W. R., & Rollnick, S. (1991). *Motivational interviewing: Preparing people to change addictive behavior.* New York: Guilford.

Miller, W. R., & Rollnick, S. (2002). What is motivational interviewing? In W. R. Miller & S. Rollnick (Eds.), *Motivational interviewing: Preparing people for change* (2nd ed., pp. 33–42). New York: Guilford.

Miller, W. K., & Rollnick, S. (2004). Talking oneself into change: Motivational interviewing, stages of change, and therapeutic process. *Journal of Cognitive Psychotherapy, 18*(4), 299–308.

Morris, J. N. (1975). *Uses of epidemiology*. New York: Churchill Livingstone.

Mossey, J. M., Mutran, E., Knott, K., & Craik, R. (1989). Determinants of recovery 12 months after hip fracture: The importance of psychosocial factors. *American Journal of Public Health, 79*, 279–286.

Moyer, A., Finney, J. W., Swearingen, C. E., & Vergun, P. (2002). Brief interventions for alcohol problems: A meta-analytic review of controlled investigations in treatment-seeking. *Addiction, 97*, 279–292.

Moyers, T. B., Martin, T., Christopher, P. J., Houck, J. M., Tonigan, J. S., & Amrhein, P. C. (2007). Client language as a mediator of motivational interviewing efficacy: Where is the evidence? *Alcoholism: Clinical and Experimental Research, 31*, 40S–47S.

Mullins, L. L., & Olson, R. A. (1990). Familial factors in the etiology, maintenance, and treatment of somatoform disorders in children. *Family Systems Medicine, 8*, 159–175.

Mussell, M., Kroenke, K., Spitzer, R. L., Williams, J. B. W., Herzog, W., & Lowe, B. (2008). Gastrointestinal symptoms in primary care: Prevalence and association with depression and anxiety. *Psychosomatic Research, 64*, 605–612.

Myers, M. F., & Gabbard, G. O. (2008). *The physician as patient: A clinical handbook for mental health professionals*. Washington, DC: American Psychiatric Association.

NIAAA. (1999). Brief intervention for alcohol problems. *Alcohol Alert, 43*, 1–6.

Nichols, M. (2008). *Family therapy: Concepts and methods*. Boston: Pearson.

Noel, M., Hickner, J., Ettenhofer, T., & Gauthier, B. (1998). The high prevalence of obesity in Michigan primary care practices: An UPRNet study. *Journal of Family Practice, 47*(1), 39.

Ockene, J. K., Kristeller, J. L., Pbert, L., Hebert, J. L., Luippold, R. S., & Goldberg, R. J. (1994). The physician-delivered smoking intervention project: Can short-term interventions produce long-term effects for a general outpatient population. *Health Psychology, 13*(3), 278–281.

O'Connor, M. J., & Whaley, S. E. (2007). Brief intervention for alcohol use by pregnant women. *American Journal of Public Health, 97*(2), 252–258.

Oquendo, M. (1995). Differential diagnosis of ataque de nervios. *American Journal of Orthopsychiatry, 65*, 60–65.

Orsillo, S. M., Roemer, L., Block-Lerner, J., LeJeune, C., & Herbert, J. D. (2004). ACT with anxiety disorders. In S. C. Hayes & K. D. Strosahl (Eds.), *A practical guide to acceptance and commitment therapy* (pp. 103–132). New York: Springer.

Öst, L. G. (2008). Efficacy of the third wave of behavior therapies: A systematic review and meta-analysis. *Behavior Research and Therapy, 46*, 296–321.

Oxman, T. E., Hegel, M. T., Hull, J. G., & Dietrich, A. J. (2008). Problem-solving treatment and coping styles in primary care for minor depression. *Journal of Consulting and Clinical Psychology, 76*, 933–943.

Palmer, R. L., Birchall, H., McGrain, L., & Sullivan, V. (2002). Self-help for bulimic disorders: A randomized controlled trial comparing minimal guidance with face-to-face or telephone guidance. *British Journal of Psychiatry, 181*, 230–235.

Park, N., Peterson, C., & Seligman, M. E. P. (2004). Strengths of character and well-being. *Journal of Social and Clinical Psychology, 22*, 603–619.

Pennebaker, J. W. (1997). *Opening up: The healing power of expressing emotions*. New York: The Guilford Press.

Pennebaker, J. W., & Francis, M. E. (1996). Cognitive, emotional, and language processes in disclosure. *Cognition and Emotion, 10*, 601–626.

Peterson, J. A. (2007). Get moving! Physical activity counseling in primary care. *Journal of the American Academy of Nurse Practitioners, 19*, 349–357.

Peterson, C., & Seligman, M. E. P. (2004). *Character strengths and virtues: A handbook and classification*. New York: Oxford University Press.

Peterson, C., Seligman, M. E. P., & Vaillant, G. E. (1988). Pessimistic explanatory style is a risk factor for physical illness: A 35 year longitudinal study. *Journal of Personality and Social Psychology, 55*, 23–27.

Petrie, K. J., Booth, R., Pennebaker, J. W., Davison, K. P., & Thomas, M. (1995). Disclosure of trauma and immune response to hepatitis B vaccination programs. *Journal of Consulting and Clinical Psychology, 63*, 787–792.

Pichot, T. (2009). *Solution-focused substance abuse treatment.* New York: Routledge.

Pollak, K. I., Østbye, T., Alexander, S. C., Gradison, M., Bastian, L. A., & Brouwer, R. J. N. (2007). Empathy goes a long way in weight loss discussions. *The Journal of Family Practice, 56*(12), 1031–1036.

Poss, J., & Jezewski, M. A. (2002). The role and meaning of susto in Mexican-Americans' explanatory model of type 2 diabetes. *Medical Anthropology Quarterly, 16*, 360–377.

Prins, A., Ouimette, P., Kimerling, R., Camerond, R. P., Hugelshofer, D. F., Shaw-Hegwer, J., et al. (2004). The primary care PTSD screen (PC-PTSD): Development and operating characteristics. *International Journal of Psychiatry in Clinical Practice, 9*, 9–14.

Prochaska, J., Redding, C. A., & Evers, K. A. (2008). The transtheoretical model and stages of change. In K. Glanz, B. Rimer, & K. Viwanath (Eds.), *Health behavior and health education* (4th ed., pp. 97–121). San Francisco: Jossey-Bass.

Prochaska, J. O., Velcier, W. F., Rossi, J. S., Goldstein, M. G., Marcus, B. H., & Rakowski, W. (1994). Stages of change and decisional balance for 12 problem behaviors. *Health Psychology, 13*, 39–46.

Rankin, E. J., Adams, R. L., & Jones, H. E. (1996). Epilepsy and nonepileptic attack disorder. In R. L. Adams, O. A. Parsons, J. L. Culbertson, & S. J. Nixon (Eds.), *Neuropsychology for clinical practice: Etiology, assessment, and treatment for common neurological disorders* (pp. 131–174). Washington, DC: American Psychological Association.

Reoux, J. P., & Miller, K. (2000). Routine hospital alcohol detoxification practice compared to symptom triggered management with an objective withdrawal scale (CIWA-Ar). *American Journal of Addictions, 9*(2), 135–144.

Ringsberg, K. C., & Krantz, G. (2006). Coping with patients with medically unexplained symptoms. *Journal of Health Psychology, 11*, 107–116.

Roberts, C. B., Vines, A. I., Kaufman, J. S., & James, S. A. (2007). Cross-sectional association between perceived discrimination and hypertension in African-American men and women. *American Journal of Epidemiology, 165*, 1–9.

Robinson, P. (2005). Adapting empirically supported treatments to the primary care setting: A template for success. In W. T. O'Donohue, M. R. Byrd, N. A. Cummings, & D. Henderson (Eds.), *Behavioral integrative care: Treatments that work in the primary care setting* (pp. 53–72). New York: Routledge.

Robinson, J. D., & Baker, J. (2006). Psychological consultation and services in a general medical hospital. *Professional Psychology: Research and Practice, 37*(3), 264–267.

Robinson, J. D., & James, L. C. (2005). Assessing the patient's need for medical evaluation: A psychologist's guide. In L. C. James & R. C. Folen (Eds.), *The primary care consultant.* Washington, DC: American Psychological Association.

Robinson, R. G., Jorge, R. E., Moser, D. J., Acion, L., Solodkin, A., Small, S. L., et al. (2008). Escitalopram and problem-solving therapy for prevention of post-stroke depression. *Journal of the American Medical Association, 299*, 2391–2400.

Robinson, P., & Reiter, J. (2007). *Behavioral consultation and primary care: A guide to integrating services.* New York: Springer.

Rollnick, S., Miller, W. R., & Butler, C. C. (2008). *Motivational interviewing in health care.* New York: Guilford.

Rosal, M. C., Ockene, J. K., Hurley, T. G., & Reiff, S. (2000). Prevalence and co-occurrence of high risk behaviors among high-risk drinkers in a primary care population. *Preventive Medicine, 31*, 140–147.

Roy-Byrne, P., Katon, W., Brodhead, W., Lepine, J. P., Richard, J., Brantley, P. J., et al. (1994). Subsyndromal (mixed) anxiety and depression in primary care. *Journal of General Internal Medicine, 9*, 507–512.

Ruddy, N. B., Borresen, D. A., & Gunn, W. B. (2008). *The collaborative psychotherapist: Creating reciprocal relationships with medical professionals.* Washington, DC: American Psychological Association.

Rural Policy Research Institute. (2008). *RUPRI data brief: Racial and ethnic composition of the population,* http://www.rupri.org/forms/race_ethnicity.pdf.

Rush, J. A., Polatin, P., & Gatchel, R. J. (2000). Depression and chronic low back pain: Establishing priorities in treatment. *Spine, 25*, 2566–2571.

Russell, M. (1994). New assessment tools for risk drinking during pregnancy. *Alcohol Health & Research World, 18*, 55–61.

Salmela, S., Poskiparta, M., Kasila, K., Vahasarja, K., & Vanhala, M. (2008). Transtheoretical model-based dietary interventions in primary care: A review of the evidence in diabetes. *Health Education Research, 24*(2), 237–252.

Scott, J. G., Cohen, D., DiCicco-Bloom, B., Orzano, J., Jaen, C. R., & Crabtree, B. F. (2001). Antibiotic use in acute respiratory infections and the ways patients pressure physicians for a prescription. *Journal of Family Practice, 10*, 853–858.

Seaburn, D. B., Lorenz, A. D., Gunn, W. B., Gawinski, B. A., & Mauksch, L. B. (1996). *Models of collaboration: A guide for mental health professionals working with health care practitioners.* New York: Basic Books.

Searight, H. R. (1992). Screening for alcohol abuse in primary care. *Family Practice Research Journal, 12*, 193–204.

Searight, H. R. (1999). *Behavioral medicine: A primary care approach.* Philadelphia: Taylor & Francis.

Searight, H. R. (2007). Efficient counseling techniques for the primary care physician. *Primary Care Clinics in Office Practice, 34*, 551–570.

Searight, H. R. (2009). Realistic approaches to counseling in the office setting. *American Family Physician, 79*(4), 277–284.

Searight, H. R., & Gafford, J. (2005). Cultural diversity at the end of life: Issues and guidelines for family physicians. *American Family Physician, 71*, 512–522.

Searight, H. R., & Gafford, J. (2006). The international medical graduate and behavioral science education. *Academic Medicine, 81*, 164–170.

Searight, H. R., & McLaren, L. (1998). Attention-deficit/hyperactivity disorder: The medicalization of misbehavior. *Journal of Clinical Psychology in Medical Settings, 5*(4), 467–495.

Searight, H. R., Price, J. W., & Gafford, J. (2004). Establishing and maintaining a psychological practice in primary care. In L. Haas (Ed.), *Handbook of primary care psychology* (4th ed.). New York: Oxford University Press.

Searight, H. R., & Searight, B. K. (2009). Working with foreign language interpreters: Recommendations for psychological practice. *Professional Psychology: Research and Practice, 40*, 444–451.

Seeman, M. V. (2008). Cross-cultural evaluation of maternal competence in a culturally diverse society. *American Journal of Psychiatry, 165*, 565–568.

Seligman, M. E. P. (1995). The effectiveness of psychotherapy: The consumer reports study. *American Psychologist, 50*, 965–974.

Seligman, M. E. P. (2002). *Authentic Happiness.* New York: The Free Press.

Seligman, M. E. P., Steen, T. A., Park, N., & Peterson, C. (2005). Positive psychology progress: Empirical validation of interventions. *American Psychologist, 60*, 410–421.

Selzer, M. L. (1971). Michigan alcohol screening test: The quest for a new diagnostic instrument. *American Journal of Psychiatry, 127*, 1653–1658.

Simkin, L. R., & Gross, A. M. (1994). Assessment of coping with high-risk situations for exercise relapse among healthy women. *Health Behavior, 13*, 274–277.

Skinner, H. A. (1982). The drug abuse screening test. *Addictive Behavior, 7*, 363–371.

Smith, S. S., Jorenby, D. E., Fiore, M. C., Anderson, J. E., Mielke, M. M., Beach, K. E., et al. (2000). Strike while the iron is hot: Can stepped-care treatments resurrect relapsed smokers? *Journal of Consulting and Clinical Psychology, 69*(3), 429–439.

Snow, L. (1993). *Walkin' over medicine.* Boulder, CO: Westview Press.

Snowden, L. R., Masland, M., & Guerrero, R. (2006). Federal civil rights policy and mental health treatment access for persons with limited English proficiency. *American Psychologist, 62*, 109–117.

Sobell, M. B., & Sobell, L. C. (2000). Stepped care as a heuristic approach to the treatment of alcohol problems. *Journal of Consulting and Clinical Psychology, 68*, 573–579.

Spitzer, R. L., Williams, J. B. W., Kroenke, K., Linzer, M., de Gruy, F. V., Hahn, S., et al. (1994). Utility of a new procedure for diagnosing mental disorders in primary care: The PRIME 1000 study. *Journal of the American Medical Association, 272*(22), 1749–1756.

Starr, P. (1982). *The social transformation of American medicine.* New York: Basic.

Stein, H. F. (1982). The annual cycle and the cultural nexus of health care behavior among Oklahoma wheat farming families. *Culture, Medicine, and Psychiatry, 6*, 81–99.

Stein, H. F. (1986). 'Sick people' and 'trolls': A contribution to the understanding of the dynamics of physician explanatory models. *Culture, Medicine, and Psychiatry, 10*, 221–229.

Stein, H. F. (1993). *American medicine as culture.* Boulder, CO: Westview Press.

Strosahl, K. D. (2005). Training behavioral health and primary care providers for integrated care: A core competencies approach. In W. T. O'Dononue, M. R. Bryd, N. A. Cummings, & D. Henderson (Eds.), *Behavioral integrative care: Treatments that work in primary care settings.* New York: Brunner-Routledge.

Strosahl, K., & Robinson, P. (2008). The primary care behavioral health model: Applications to prevention, acute care and chronic management. In R. K. D. Stafford (Ed.), *Collaborative medicine case studies: Evidence in practice.* New York: Springer.

Stuart, M. R., & Lieberman, J. A. (2008). *The 15 minute hour: Therapeutic talk in primary care.* New York: Radcliffe Publishing.

Sullivan, J. T., Sykora, K., Schneiderman, J., Naranjo, C. A., & Sellers, E. M. (1989). Assessment of alcohol withdrawal: The revised Clinical Institute Withdrawal Assessment for Alcohol Scale (CIWA-Ar). *British Journal of Addictions, 84*, 1353–1357.

Susser, E. S., & Schwartz, S. (2006). Diversity of cohort studies. In S. Susser, E. S. Schwartz, A. Morabia, & E. J. Bromet (Eds.), *Psychiatric epidemiology* (pp. 108–137). New York: Oxford.

Tate, D. F., Jackvony, E. H., & Wing, R. R. (2003). Effects of internet behavioral counseling in weight loss in adults at risk for type 2 diabetes. *Journal of the American Medical Association, 289*(14), 1833–1836.

Taylor, R. L. (2007). *Psychological masquerade: Distinguishing psychological from organic disorders.* New York: Springer.

Taylor, S., Sirois, F., & Tripp, D. (2009). *Health psychology.* New York: McGraw-Hill.

Tillman, R., & Geller, B. (2005). A brief screening tool for a prepubertal and early adolescent bipolar disorder phenotype. *American Journal of Psychiatry, 162*, 1214–1216.

Tolin, D. F., Diefenbach, G. J., Maltby, N., & Hannan, S. (2005). Stepped care for obsessive-compulsive disorder: A pilot study. *Cognitive Behavioral Practice, 12*, 403–414.

Tukel, R., Polat, A., Ozdemir, O., Aksut, D., & Turksoy, N. (2002). Comorbid conditions in obsessive-compulsive disorder. *Comprehensive Psychiatry, 43*, 204–209.

Van Melle, J. P., de Jonge, P., Spijkerman, T. A., Tijssen, J. G. P., Ormel, J., van Veldhuisen, D. J., et al. (2004). Prognostic association of depression following myocardial infarction with mortality and cardiovascular events: A meta-analysis. *Psychosomatic Medicine, 66*, 814–822.

Wagner, H. R., Burns, B. J., Broadhead, W. E., Yarnall, K. S. H., Sigmon, A., & Gaynes, B. N. (2000). Minor depression in family practice: Functional morbidity, comorbidity, service utilization and outcomes. *Psychological Medicine, 30*, 1377–1390.

Waskett, C. (1999). Confidentiality in a team setting. In R. Bor & D. McCann (Eds.), *The practice of counseling in primary care* (pp. 118–139). London: Sage.

Webster. (2002). *A history of the national health service.* New York: Oxford.

Wedding, D., & Mengel, M. (2004). Models of integrated care in primary care settings. In L. Haas (Ed.), *Handbook of Primary Care Psychology* (pp. 47–61). New York: Oxford.

Weiss, G., & Hechtman, L. (1993). *Hyperactive children grown up.* New York: Guilford.

White, M. (1995). *Re-authoring lives: Interviews and essays.* Adelaide, Australia: Dulwich Center Publications.

Wilk, A. I., Jensen, N. M., & Havighurst, T. C. (1997). Meta-analysis of randomized controlled trials addressing brief interventions in heavy alcohol drinkers. *Journal of General Internal Medicine, 12*, 274–283.

Williams, J. W., Barret, J., Oxman, T., Frank, E., Katon, W., & Sullivan, M. (2000). Treatment of dysthymia and minor depression in primary care. *Journal of the American Medical Association, 284*, 1519–1526.

Witkiewitz, K., & Marlatt, G. A. (2004). Relapse prevention for alcohol and drug problems: That was Zen, this is Tao. *American Psychologist, 59*(4), 224–235.

Wood, M. E., Stockdale, A., & Flynn, B. S. (2008). Interviews with primary care physicians regarding taking and interpreting the cancer family history. *Family Practice, 25*, 334–340.

World Health Organization. (2003). *Adult self-report scale-VI.I (ASRS-VI.I).*

World Health Organization. (2006). *Constitution of the World Health Organization,* http://www.who.int/governance/eb/who_constitution_en.pdf. (Downloaded September 12, 2009).

Yalom, I. D. (1995). *Theory and practice of group psychotherapy* (4th ed.). New York: Basic.

Yalom, I. D., & Leszcz, M. (2005). *Theory and practice of group psychotherapy* (5th ed.). New York: Basic.

Yesavage, J. A., Brink, T. L., Rose, T. L., Lum, O., Huanag, V., Adey, M., et al. (1983). Development and validation of a geriatric depression screening scale: A preliminary report. *Journal of Psychiatric Research, 17*, 37–49.

Yick, A. G., & Gupta, R. (2002). Chinese cultural dimensions of death, dying and bereavement: Focus group findings. *Journal of Cultural Diversity, 9*, 32–42.

Zimmerman, R., Ahsan, H., & Susser, E. (2006). Modern family history studies. In E. S. Susser, S. Schwartz, A. Morabia, & E. J. Bromet (Eds.), *Psychiatric epidemiology.* New York: Oxford.

Index

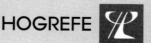

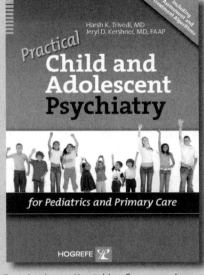
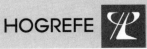

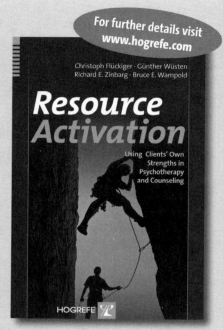
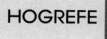